feel fab at ZPL

feel fab at 52

Sue Donnelly

First Published In Great Britain 2008
by www.BookShaker.com

© Copyright Sue Donnelly

Typeset in Trebuchet

I dedicate this book to all my wonderful teachers who have supported, inspired and educated me in my journey thus far.

Jennifer Aston
Suzy Greaves
Kim Bolsover
Gerina Gaffney
Evana Maggiore
Rosemarie Williams
Debbie Gray
Carla Mathis
Caroline Harbord
Pippa Rees
Laura Howard
Brenda Kinsel
Caroline Moroz
Andrea Kwiatkowski
Sue Clarke
Jo Parfitt
Tony Mayer
Damien Churton
Paula Gardner
Nick Williams
Julia Brown

And my fabulous clients who have allowed me to help them realise how gorgeous they really are.

Thank you!

Contents

Praise for Sue's Advice

"As the parent to two gorgeous teenage girls who turn heads, I went to see Sue feeling mumsy and invisible. After years of trial and error I was generally dressing to suit my shape but tended to pick the same things over and over again. Although my clothes were expensive I felt that I definitely lacked the wow factor. Sue immediately made me feel good by telling me I was really pretty as I walked in her front door. I haven't heard that for quite a while and she even said - a little later - that had a nice bottom and I haven't heard that for over 20 years! Sue has made me realize that even in 'middle age' I can look attractive and sexy. My confidence has definitely increased and as soon as I got home I followed her specific advice and went and bought a stretchy pencil skirt that I have barely taken off since. It looks fab."

Jenny - Solicitor

"At RSVP Introductions we find Sue's style guidance invaluable. Her relaxed yet unfailingly upbeat style has helped many of our clients over 45 gain their confidence when they find themselves back on the dating scene after a long relationship. One said to me just the other day, after a date arranged through us, 'And I looked pretty hot I must say - thanks to Sue.'"

Anne - Director RSVP Introductions

"I no longer buy black and my wardrobe looks a whole lot better for it! I have just replaced my glasses and after wearing them for 30 years this was the first time I made my choice with confidence - and enjoyed doing so too. I no longer consider what size I should buy, but pick the one that looks best. It is very liberating when you know what suits you - no longer worry about whether things are in fashion, just whether they look good."

Clare - Head of HR

"I first got in touch with Sue when approaching my 50th birthday. I had lost all confidence in my appearance and actually dreaded clothes shopping because I felt nothing ever looked good. Sue turned this negative attitude around in one session! Since then I have also attended her Heading South course which was really informative and so much fun. I have also recommended Sue to several friends and their feedback to me is always about the impact Sue's advice and positivity has had on their confidence and attitude to their appearance at this important time of our lives. Equally important is her none threatening approach – it's like going shopping with a really knowledgeable good friend who genuinely wants you to look your best."

Steph - Manager

"Approaching my forties and feeling frumpy, old-fashioned and having a poor body image was not a good role model for my daughters. If I felt like this at 40 and did nothing about it, how would I feel at 50? I booked a long overdue consultation with Sue. Her friendly and down to earth advice gave me the confidence to try new styles and colours which I previously would not have considered wearing. I have never had so few clothes and yet so much to wear! My meeting Sue was one of the best things I have ever done and has changed my life. Having gained new found confidence in this area has given me confidence in other areas of my life too - she is a wonderful teacher and I will never forget what she did for me."

Sarah - Mum and Company Director's Wife

"If you are wondering whether to ask Sue to go through your wardrobe and discuss your style, please do not wait a moment longer. First, you find out what not to wear and although this term had been popular for some time it is only now that I fully realize how important it is. It saves you looking round three quarters of each store and allows you to concentrate on what to wear. You are then very focused and clear about what to wear. The 'templates' and tips Sue sends you remind you of the styles that suit and instead of standing in stores looking aimlessly and helplessly round, you can hone directly in on what you need. Sue encouraged me to try different stores and taught me that I needn't always spend money. In fact one of the unexpected things to happen after the session is that I have only spent a small amount of money but have a lot of outfits. In terms of revelations, I can wear a belt and I have short legs! How did I spend 48 years not knowing this? I would recommend this session to every woman who wants the confidence to leave the house knowing she looks the best she can and who wants to take the fear and anxiety out of choosing clothes."

Gillian

"A very big thank you for carefully escourting me on a journey of rediscovery, the subject matter was a very fragile 'me' and sadly more than a little wanting in most areas. You helped me evaluate myself, to build on the assets that for a long time I had forgotten I had and best of all discover some that I had never seen before. Presenting to me my colour palette and how to use it has given me back the confidence that is all too often lost when one becomes a mother, not that I would ever change the latter. In short, you have been that inexpensive discovery that has made me feel the richest woman on earth. A huge thank you Sue."

Ruth Foreman

Foreword

For almost ten years now, since I first realized the link between environment and empowerment through my study of the ancient Chinese philosophy of Feng Shui, my personal mission has been to restore sacredness to the everyday act of getting dressed. Clothing is your body's most intimate environment, and therefore as influential on the quality of your existence as according to Feng Shui, are your home and work decors. Your clothes both reflect who you are and attract what you will be, do and have. You are, and you become, what you wear... no matter what your age!

When this book was in its planning stages, Sue Donnelly began to approach influential women 'of a certain age' to invite them to participate in this project. For once, I felt blessed to be a fifty-something. Sue's enthusiasm for this subject, herself on the verge of joining the Half-Century Club, was contagious, and I eagerly awaited the arrival of her *Feel Fab at 50* manuscript. I was not disappointed. I just wish I was a few years younger so this chock-full of inner and outer wisdom book could have ushered me into 'middle age'.

Sue's delightfully honest and humorous writing style and sage fashion and beauty advice truly pays homage to her expertise. An industry recognised author and internationally acclaimed image consultant, Sue also has the honour of being the United Kingdom's first (and at the time of this writing, the only,) certified Fashion Feng Shui® Facilitator. Or, should I say that I have the honour of having Sue Donnelly be the first to represent my transformational dressing technique 'across the pond'. I cannot think of anyone who more aligns with the vision that I hold for, and the integrity that is, Fashion Feng Shui®.

So, to all you SASSY (Sensational, Assured, Sensual/Sexy, Stimulating and Youthful) women out there, buckle your seat belts before you continue with this book, because Sue Donnelly is going to take you on the 'read' of your life!

Evana Maggiore, AICI, CIP
Founder and President of Fashion Feng Shui® International, LLC
Author of 'Fashion Feng Shui: The Power of Dressing with Intention'
www.fashionfengshui.com

Curiosity Killed The Cat (or Did It?)

"Clothes maketh the man. Naked people have little or no influence in society."

MARK TWAIN

It's not every day you wake up to the realisation that you share something very special with Madonna... and Michelle Pfeiffer, Sharon Stone, Kate Bush, Anita Baker, Annette Bening, Holly Hunter, Ellen De Generes, Jamie Lee Curtis and Andie MacDowell to name but a few. Celebrity, good looks, fame and fortune – great if it were true, but no. What is it we have in common? We were all 1958 babies so we're all celebrating 50th birthdays this year.

Many years ago, turning 50 would have been a sign that you were definitely in 'middle age'. The permed hair, loose comfortable clothing and looking forward to having grandchildren would have been nothing out of the ordinary. These days we expect something totally different and sometimes it's hard to define exactly what that is. We don't want to dress like our mothers but we certainly don't want to look like our daughter's twin sister either.

In other cultures, older women are highly respected and revered for their wisdom and age. Here in the UK this tradition seems to have died a death. Old is old and youth is the new black. The celebrities mentioned earlier look younger than their years, slim, confident and successful, so the pressure is on us to conform to their stereotype. "Why can't we look like that?" we ask ourselves. Of course, money and trappings such as the personal trainer, stylist, hairdresser, make up artist and gourmet chef enable them to stay on top of this beauty game. They also have access to cosmetic procedures, both surgical and those of a less invasive nature, if they choose to go that route but it's not always the answer. Michael Jackson also turns 50 this year and his life has not always been a happy one.

I am certainly not against plastic surgery or any procedure that can help you live your life feeling more confident and carefree. A nip and tuck in the right place can do wonders for the way you look. Cosmetic procedures can reap massive rewards if this is your only option. Loose folds of skin after multiple births, eye bags, droopy bosoms after breast feeding or a very large bust which causes tremendous back pain for instance, can make life pretty miserable for the owner and none of these can be rectified in any other way, however fit and healthy you are. Too much though, and you end up with a face that is just unreal and doesn't give any hints to who you really are. There are no guarantees with cosmetic surgery. We have all seen the horrors when it has gone hideously wrong. The 'trout pout' has been well documented in the press for a very long time.

Surgery, purely for reasons of vanity alone, can be a dangerous course of action. It can help one to look younger but it's a never-ending project. Think of painting a house. You start with the door. It looks so fresh with its new shiny coat of paint. With a sinking feeling you become aware that now the doorframe looks tired. To create balance, more maintenance work is needed. So you paint the doorframe, but once completed the poor state of the windows comes into view and so we go on. The sad fact is that emotionally, you may not actually feel any better but your bank balance will soon notice the difference. Interestingly enough, over 80% of cosmetic surgery in the UK is carried out on those of us under 50, so may be our sixth decade concentrates on acceptance and natural enhancement rather than invasion.

Botox and other non surgical procedures are well utilised but there is still a lack of real scientific evidence to say what might occur as a result of use at a later date and do you really want to lose your facial expressiveness? Many celebrities, such as Lulu, have actively stopped using these procedures as they feel they are making them appear older in the long run.

Many celebrities maintain a very restrictive diet to keep their slim shape but there can be health risks involved with this, especially with the desire to become a size zero. I myself had eating disorders for a number of years, and though I lived to tell the tale, my body still shows the scars. It's not about punishing yourself in a physical sense either, as the type of exercise programme we need in later life differs dramatically to that of a younger person, especially if you're going through the menopause.

So this book is not about any of those things, though I may touch on them. This book is about how you can make the most of your physical attributes, naturally, using clothes to actively highlight your assets and to disguise the bits you're not so keen on.

For me, turning 50 meant many things. For one, and I know it's a little morbid, I've had to come to terms with the fact that I have now walked on this planet for more than half of my life. I realise that I have done many things in the past which have not served me well, either physically or emotionally. I expect you have too – it's called 'living'. Any 0 year is a turning point and 50 is no different in that respect. However, its occurrence has spurred me on to make sure that I live the best life I can, one that fulfils and sustains me, while I'm also looking and feeling fabulous too.

Like most women my age I sometimes look in the mirror and am horrified at what I see. The youthful girl inside of me is totally incongruent with the reflection staring back at me. My bodily parts appear to have drifted south without my noticing. My clients, though different in nature, all seem to share the same concerns and their questions to me are along the following lines:

"Why do I look so tired all the time?"

"What can I do to hide my thighs/stomach/droopy knees?"

"How come my eyes look piggy?"

"How much longer do I need to dye my hair?"

"Can I really get way with wearing this?"

"Will I look like mutton dressed as lamb?"

"I'm scared the younger shop assistants will stare at me if try anything on."

"I feel so frumpy/fat/skinny, what can I do?"

"Is this it?"

All of the above can be solved. Really.

As a 'middle aged' Image Coach, I will share with you what I have learned, for no longer do we have to look as though we're 'past it'. In fact the stereotypical older woman, who traditionally has been abandoned by her husband for a younger model, is disappearing fast. In her place has evolved a new type of 50 year old. She is the one more likely to leave, often replacing her husband with a toy boy because an older man just can't keep up with her or, more frequently, choosing to remain happily single. Recent research by the University of Kent has said that women finally admit they are old when they have reached 72, whereas men believe old age begins at 55. As the population of the UK gets older, what we term as middle age is taking a dramatic shift upwards.

If you're in your 40s though, you may be struggling a little to come to terms with ageing and all that goes with it. In the UK, 44 is the age where most females feel at their lowest ebb. The good thing is that most women over 50 are at their happiest, so it's really important to bridge that gap and that's where this book comes in.

This is the first time in history we have managed to add years to our age but remain under-developed in our minds. In the past, people had to grow old more quickly as they needed to mature to cope with the ravages of wartime. We have not had to do that. As a result, we have been given the gift of an extra 20 years in which to grow and flourish. These additional years aren't piled on at the end of our lives when we reach 70 or 80 but instead we need to utilise them in our 'middle' ages. It would be a shame to waste them.

If you are ready to make some positive changes to the way you look, increasing your confidence and making heads turn, then this book is for you. A daily newspaper recently used the term WOW – Wealthy, Older Women – and that's fine if it's what you want from life. I feel there is more to it than that. Why can't we be SASSY – Sensational, Assured, Sensual/Sexy, Stimulating and Youthful too?

This book will help you to learn how to feel good and look great when your body is fighting the laws of gravity. Dwelling on how you used to look isn't helpful when you may still have another 30 years or more to live. Feeling down about yourself will drain your confidence and prevent you from living at your peak potential. On the other hand, when you look good, you feel good and your self-esteem increases. In turn, this will enable you to project yourself with more conviction and confidence. Others are drawn to you, so you are likely to gain more positive responses from work associates, family, friends and even strangers. And guess what; your confidence (and your positive attitude to everything you do) increases even more.

Dressing in the same way as you did 20 years ago isn't going to do you any favours. Neither are your makeup and hair if you haven't changed them in decades. Yes, your body has most definitely gone through many changes and it's difficult to turn back the clock, so you need to know what to do right now.

What this book doesn't set out to do is change the intrinsic you. Your "self" is what you are all about. Just because you're older doesn't mean you have to adopt a new personality. Its aim is to show you how to dress in a way that reflects your core essence and your personal intentions as well as your shape and your lifestyle. Remaining authentic is crucial if you want to truly align your image and the impact you make with your personal values. As Annie Morrow Lindbergh said, "The most exhausting thing you can be is inauthentic". Just because something looks good on your friend does not mean it will look good on you.

Many of us are time poor so you don't need to read this book in one long sitting. Choose the chapter that resonates with you and start there. Begin to put each lesson into practice when you have the time to do so properly. Everything in this book is easily do-able without resorting to surgery or other cosmetic procedures, though that choice is available if you wish to include it.

Something you might want to think about when you read this book is your own journey and how you tackle it so it serves you in the very best possible way. After each chapter I have included Words of Wisdom that you might want to ponder. Use these and the accompanying exercises to log your own observations, thoughts and feelings.

I rarely make New Year's Resolutions as I believe most of them are discarded by the middle of January, creating guilt and a feeling of failure. What I do instead is choose a word that sums up exactly how I want the year to pan out. This year my word is 'curiosity'. To demonstrate what I mean, the word I chose for last year was 'peachy'. I wanted a year that was juicy, fuzzy, warm and full of sun. I got it. Being curious means that I act as an observer of my actions rather than becoming judgmental. It denotes playfulness rather than rigidity. There is no guilt attached to my failings, as being curious allows me to say to myself "So, that's what happens when I..." I urge you to try it. Make a note of your own personal word right now.

Turning 50 does not mean you have to deny the child within. Recognising playfulness and joy is what youthfulness is all about. So part of this book will be about my curiosity and my own journey's observations as I certainly don't have all the answers – or not yet anyway. So laugh along with me at my 'disasters' and learn from my successes and don't get alarmed if you have some dodgy moments of your own.

My aim is to serve my clients in the best way I know how. As I will not meet most of you face to face, I really hope you enjoy the book and, more importantly, this wonderful time of your life. Please accept the knowledge and training I have accumulated and recorded in this book as my gift to you. I hope you find it useful, practical, thought provoking and totally transformational. Here's to SASSY women everywhere.

Sue Donnelly
June 2008

Mind Over Matter
(Beauty & The Beast)

"It may sound like a cliché, but beauty for me really does start on the inside. It's like a state of mind, a state of love if you will. Then, whatever you can do on the outside is all like a bonus."

QUEEN LATIFAH

These days reaching so called 'middle age' no longer needs to stereotype us as old women. I have met all sorts of women in their 40s and 50s with completely different lifestyles. We can be new mums or empty nesters, company directors/high earning executives or homemakers, divorced/widowed or new to marriage, mature students or retired from work and so on. We are all different and that is what is so marvellous about being middle aged *now*.

But sadly, many of us do seem to have something in common. We no longer feel attractive and/or we have lost all sense of how to dress ourselves to look phenomenal.

Wouldn't it be great if we could have an angel wave a magic wand over us and suddenly we know we are drop dead gorgeous? Or better still, we're presented with our own personal stylist. You may not be able to afford the latter and even wishful thinking won't enable an angel to materialise but it doesn't mean that you can't be beautiful in your own unique way.

1

What is beauty anyway? They say that 'beauty is in the eye of the beholder' but is it?

I often carry out small surveys of my own (being curious, of course), amongst friends and clients. This time I chose both sexes and a variety of age groups. The results:

The qualities of an attractive woman:

- ✓ confidence
- ✓ happiness
- ✓ charisma
- ✓ authenticity

No mention of long blonde hair or big boobs, long legs or flawless skin. In fact some of the men I spoke to detested the 'plastic' look of someone who had received cosmetic surgery. It was more to do with someone feeling comfortable in their own skin, thus giving energy and purpose to their lives and those of other people. No one was captivated by self-absorption, self denial (of food, clothing or any other aspect of nurturing), obsession with one's own body/looks or a sense of selfishness either. A person's spirit definitely can add or detract to the notion of beauty and attractiveness.

Unfortunately, most of us dwell on what we lack, rather than the assets we have, thinking it will make people think better of us. We know it's not 'British' to boast but even the most glamorous celebrities bemoan their appearance. The press has quoted Michelle Pfeiffer as saying that she walks like a duck, Nigella Lawson doesn't like her 'sticky out stomach' and Madonna doesn't want her 'fat, Italian thighs' photographed. It seems no one is immune from this constant pressure to look perfect, however beautiful we think they are.

The mind is very strong and it chatters incessantly so we end up believing what it says. I label these negative thoughts and beliefs 'the beast' and it resides within all of us. All of us have parts of our bodies that we don't love very much and the beast makes sure we never forget:

"You can't wear that with your thighs!"

"You look ridiculous in that outfit."

"Look at those wrinkles."

The beast is relentless. We've suffered years of backchat and now believe every word it says is the gospel truth. What we forget is that whatever figure faults we may think we have are usually compensated by something that another person would give their eye teeth to own. For instance, if you have a large tum, odds are you'll have a great bum. Large boobs and a short waist usually sit with long legs. Shorter legs often go hand in hand with a long body and a flat tum. A wrinkled face may belong to a slim body whereas a plumper body can often result in younger looking skin. So turn your attention to the assets you have. It's highly likely that no-one else will even be aware of your hang ups but the more you draw attention to your challenges by talking about them, the more others will begin to notice. Be aware of your problem areas and cover them up by all means, but don't forget to showcase your assets.

We all owe it to ourselves to recognise how absolutely fabulous we are – I know it may be difficult but, trust me, you are beautiful in your own right and I need you to know that.

I spoke earlier about a journey so you may want to make a record of what happens to you along the way. If so, I would suggest you buy a really beautiful journal to inspire and motivate you. Any old notebook just will not do for someone as gorgeous as you.

Step 1: I would like you to take a good, long look at yourself in a full-length mirror. If you can manage to do this without wearing any clothes, even better.

Step 2: Let's get the negative stuff out of the way. Write down ten things you don't like about yourself. I know ten sounds a lot but I expect the beast will help you along and you'll do it in no time at all.

Things I don't like about myself:

....

....

....

....

....

....

....

....

....

....

Step 3: Put a large X through them.

I'm not saying they are unimportant but you don't need to dwell on them, just be aware of their existence. You also need to shut your beast up once and for all and this is a great first step to doing that.

Step 4: Write down five things that you like about yourself. They don't have to be major. It could be you like your blue eyes, or you have small well-shaped feet. Just be positive about it. This may take a little longer but please persevere. It will be worth it in the end.

....

....

....

....

....

Step 5: Now, write down a further five things you like about yourself. I know this might be hard but PLEASE do it. Take a really long look at yourself, not a cursory glance. Look at your body as though you had never seen it before. Be curious. What can you discover about yourself?

....

....

....

....

....

Step 6: I want you to imagine that you are falling in love. If you have a partner already, is he or she perfect in the way they look? What attracts you to them? Write it down.

Odds are they are not perfect but they are still attractive, sexy and fanciable. They may have some quirkiness in their features which really turns you on. It makes them different and forms part of their charm. Do you see, you don't have to be perfect; you just have to allow yourself to be you. So what if you have a lop-sided face – it's what makes you, you. Look at it and love it. It allows you to smile and laugh and show pleasure and connect with others. How wonderful is that?

Imagine you are getting married to yourself. Think about the vows you would make, to love, honour and cherish yourself from this day forth. Please do this for yourself. This means treating yourself as someone special all the time.

See yourself as an entire being, a whole person. I hear so many women saying, "I hate my stomach" or similar remarks on a regular basis. They are so hard on themselves. We are more than just one offending body part. Try to love all of yourself in equal measure. Touch your stomach, your thigh, or whatever you don't like and be kind to it. Anoint it with beautiful creams or oils, take care of it like you would a child. Your body has been through many things – given birth and suckled a child maybe - so treat it with reverence and respect. Without a functioning body, we can do nothing. Because of the power of our mind, which wants to be in control at all times, most of us see our body as a separate part of ourselves instead of a wonderful piece of our whole being.

If you receive a compliment about the way you look, I want you to accept it. No more replies such as "this old thing" or "it only cost…" Imagine the compliment as a box of your favourite chocolates or a bouquet of flowers. Would you throw them back to the person giving them to you? Of course you wouldn't. Not accepting a compliment is just as rude. You are in effect saying that the giver has no judgment or taste. Practise saying "thank you". Nothing more, nothing less, just "thank you" until it feels very comfortable to do so.

Step 7: To keep you motivated, I would like you to think of a positive affirmation about yourself. It must be written with the 3 Ps in mind:

- ✓ Personal
- ✓ Present Tense
- ✓ Positive

For example, "I'm a sexy siren and men find me captivating" or "I am adored for my beauty and wisdom" or "My sense of fun distinguishes me from the rest."

You will need to find something that really resonates with you. It's no good using the word sexy if you don't want to feel that way. Perhaps chic and stylish would be a better fit. It may be that you have to look to the past. Did you feel more special in days gone by? What's changed? How can you recapture it? Try a few out until you find the one that really harmonises with what you want to be.

My Affirmation is:

....

....

....

....

....

....

....

....

....

....

Practise saying it out loud to yourself in the mirror. Write it down on several pieces of card. Place them so can't miss them wherever you go – in your purse, on the fridge, in the bathroom mirror and so on. If this is inappropriate, if you share with others for example, then keep it in your handbag or in your underwear drawer but it must be somewhere you visit at least once a day.

Step 8: Keep noticing how you feel and make notes in your beautiful journal. Has anyone treated you differently? Has the beast gone away yet? Catch yourself in conversation with the beast and say, "you're wrong." You have no further use for its negativity. Step outside yourself and see it for what it is - a menace.

Personalise the beast by giving it a name. Mine's called Fred and when we have our conversations, I listen to him and then I say, "Fred, those are your opinions, not mine. I am quite capable of making my own mind up, thank you."

If, like me, you have a mind that rarely switches off, it can be more effective to write to your beast instead. If I am feeling particularly low, I write down all the things I think I can't do, for instance, 'I can't wear that dress as my legs are too fat'. I then go through the letter, cross out all reference to 'I' and change it to 'Fred says'. When Fred says I can't wear it because my legs are too fat, my immediate reaction is, "I'll show him," and I usually do.

Step 9: Keep your journal by your bedside, and every night write down three nice things that have happened to you that day. Even if it's a smile and hello from a relative stranger it's worth noting down. Call it your Gratitude Page. When you have positive things on your mind just before sleeping, you'll find yourself in a more positive frame of mind in the morning. Watch how these increase over the next few weeks in both frequency and power. You'll be amazed at how your gratitude pages keep growing.

Step 10: Read this book.

You have now begun in earnest and taken your biggest step forward. The rest will be easy. Let the book show you how to embrace your best qualities and dress them to your advantage. Show off your personality and celebrate your uniqueness. I want you to. There is only one you and the world needs you to be your most fabulous self. There is no dress rehearsal in life, so make the most of the one you've got now, before it's too late.

WORDS OF WISDOM

✓ Try not to see yourself as separate body parts. You are a unique and beautiful person so cherish the bits of you that you would normally loathe.

✓ Perfection is unattainable so don't beat yourself up about it. Do the best you can and enjoy the results.

✓ Don't compare yourself to anyone else – there's no point.

✓ Don't forget that others may well be envious of you.

✓ Don't hide your light under a bushel.

Build a Secure Foundation

"Brevity is the soul of lingerie."

DOROTHY PARKER

A house needs the correct foundations to remain upright and secure (whatever the weather) and your body is no different. The wrong underpinnings can ruin an outfit instantly, however much it cost. Spend time and money on selecting the right size and style of undergarments and instantly transform your shape. The added bonus is that you may lose pounds in the process.

The prettier the underwear, the less practical it is. Lace can look 'bumpy' under fine fabrics. Keep it for the bedroom and wear plain, seamless bras to maintain a sleek silhouette. This may mean purchasing a strapless, a balcony, a seamless and a push-up bra, though a convertible one, which has many ways of fastening the straps, is a very useful addition to your lingerie drawer. Don't buy too many bras as most of us tend to wear the same ones until they become grey and the rest remain untouched. The shelf life of a bra is only four months if regularly washed. After sixteen weeks, wear and tear will mean that the bra is no longer supporting your breasts properly.

We spend in excess of £640 million on bras but 80% of women are wearing the wrong size. Your nipples should sit halfway between your neck and your waist so have a look in the mirror and check the placement of your breasts.

If you have large breasts, it is essential that you have yourself measured correctly, probably every six months. Manufacturers' sizings can differ widely so don't think because you are a 36D in one bra that you are a 36D in another. Department stores can have up to 40 suppliers for their lingerie, so sizing is bound to differ.

Bras that fit badly not only look horrendous, especially if flesh is spilling out over the cups, but can also promote sagging of the breast tissue and stretch marks. If that wasn't enough, the wrong size bra can cause headaches, cysts, neck ache and back ache.

The average size of a woman's breast has increased over the years to an E/F cup. As a result, you'll find a much wider selection of larger cup sizes than in previous years. Rigby & Peller (*www.rigbyandpeller.com*) and Bravissimo (*www.bravissimo.com*) offer bras that are sexy even in very large sizes. M&S have just introduced a J cup so expect other stores to follow suit. They also stock AA for those of us at the other extreme. However small your bust, you should still wear a bra every day for support, especially if doing any sporting activity.

HOW TO MEASURE YOUR BUST

Wrap a soft tape measure around your ribcage, just under your bust. Add 5 inches to the measurement if it's an odd number and 6 if it's even. This is your band size.

Next, take a loose measurement across the fullest part of your bust. The difference between the two measurements is your cup size as follows:

A	=	1"
B	=	2"
C	=	3"
D	=	4"
DD	=	5"
DDD	=	6"

If you're larger than this, I advise going for a professional fitting.

FIT

Cups: Your breasts should fill the cups completely with no overspill at the top or the sides. If the fabric wrinkles, it means the bra is too large or the wrong shape. Go down a size or try another style with more coverage. Spillage means it's too small for you. Go up a size or get one with more coverage. If your breasts are different in size, ask for specialist help or buy a 'chicken fillet' to balance the smaller side. The channels that enclose any underwiring should fully enclose the breast and lie flat. They should never sit on top of the breast tissue itself.

Straps: There should be no pinching or cutting into the shoulders and no sliding either. Adjustable straps allow for optimum fit but if they keep slipping try a racing back. If they pinch, try a more supportive style with padding.

The Band: It should fit snugly round your ribcage so you can push a finger underneath. If you can't it's too tight. It the band rides up your back it's too loose. Unsightly rolls of flesh below or above means it's far too small. The closure on the band should lie flat.

Make sure the bra is comfortable when you buy it. A bra can be very much like new shoes – if it's not comfortable in the fitting room, it certainly won't be when you're wearing it all day.

Ensure your breasts sit level with your mid upper arm and that they stay put if you lift your arms.

Mastectomy: There's no need to despair as there is lots of choice on the market today, both for pretty lingerie and fabulous swimwear. One of the best sites to look at is *www.amoena.co.uk* (tel: 0800 072 8866). They have a really great range of underwear and swimwear in cup sizes A-DD. If you have a larger bust or like the idea of a strapless top, with bra included, try *www.eloise.co.uk* with sizing up to an E cup, or *www.nicolajane.com* which goes from AA-DD. As long as the scar tissue is not damaged further by badly fitting underwiring, most women can still wear sexy bras. For the ultimate in luxury, try Rigby & Peller who have a specialist mastectomy service and the most amazing underwear. For further details ring 0207 491 2200 or go online to *www.rigbyandpeller.com*

There are many types of bra and it's important you choose the correct one for each occasion.

THE BOTTOM LINE

As we get older, our bottoms can sag so we may need some extra help. VPL (visible panty lines) are a real no-no but thongs may not always be the answer. Larger tums or bums can benefit from knickers that 'hold you in', whereas boy leg briefs or shorts are useful for those with more pert behinds. Just make sure that the waistline fits well and isn't too tight or you'll have a roll of extra flesh to contend with. I usually buy briefs that are a size larger than my normal size and this seems to work. Whatever you choose, Bridget Jones' big pants are definitely out. We're talking fabulous at 50, not frumpy!

TUMMY TROUBLE

A higher waistline coupled with strong fibres are what you need to combat problems in the tummy region. Most department stores have their own ranges in stock. Try several out until you find the one that suits your figure best. Some have control in the thigh area too. Sexy they are not, but they provide you with a fantastic silhouette if worn under a figure-hugging 'knock 'em dead' dress. Spanx is a good brand and offers a variety of different styles.

DROOPY DRAWERS

Those of us with very long bodies may find our bottom is a little too close to our knees from the rear view. If so, try *www.figleaves.com* for pants with uplift. You can even buy pads to put in your knickers to give you a J-Lo bottom if that's what you crave.

CELLULITE

Playtex and M&S have ranges which include thigh and tummy slimmers, so cellulite may appear less obvious.

If you're fuller figured go to Rigby & Peller or Bravissimo. Both have a wonderful selection of corsetry that gives freedom and control, and still makes you look gorgeous and curvy. So you can relax *and* look sexy.

John Lewis is now offering a specially tailored service for control underwear. You can book an appointment, which is free, with your local store's lingerie department.

STOCKING FILLERS

There's nothing worse than seeing a pair of lily-white, goose-bumpy legs so that's why it's a pleasure to see so many different styles of hose around. My own feeling is that I rarely wear 10 denier, tan tights unless the outfit really called for it. They're not trendy, they are prone to snagging, and getting the colour just right is a nightmare. Go for heavier and more fashionable options.

If you're like me and wear tights most of the time (a pair of hold- ups slid down my legs in the middle of a very important presentation I was giving – so never again!) you may find them tight and restrictive around the waist area. Well, problem solved. Many stores now stock a variety of 'hipster' tights with a low rise.

Woolly or ribbed tights are lovely and warm to wear. They may not seem sexy but can be made to look chic if teamed with a pair of high wedges or some sexy boots. Beware of heavily ribbed styles unless you have ultra thin legs. They can add pounds.

Patterned tights are best worn with plain clothes. The larger the pattern the less flattering to your legs. Never wear with a printed garment. Vertical stripes can lengthen the legs so are useful to the short-legged amongst us.

Colourful tights can be wonderful or ghastly. If you're young at heart, brave or both, you could try mixing colours that clash such as orange and pink. For the rest of us, match your tights to your skirt and shoes but be slightly daring with the colour you choose. Why not try olive green or deep purple? Make sure they are matt/opaque not shiny, as the latter will make your legs look bigger. I tend to jazz up my more boring neutral dresses this way. A lovely grey knit I have comes alive with purple tights and matching shoes. The bonus is my legs look really long. I team with a handbag also in purple but a different shade. Too much 'matching' is very dated and 'mumsy'.

Of course, these suggestions may not be the best thing to wear if you're expecting a night of passion but they will get you noticed and for all the right reasons.

WORDS OF WISDOM

✓ Change your underwear often so it supports you correctly.

✓ Buy lingerie according to what you will wear on top.

✓ Get measured every year.

✓ Don't forget to look at your rear view in the mirror before you go out.

✓ Don't skimp on this part of your outfit or the overall effect will be ruined.

Accentuate The Positive (How To Make The Most of Your Assets)

"Style is very different from fashion. Once you find something that works, keep it"

TOM FORD

How many times have you spotted a fabulous garment in a shop window, a magazine or on-line and gasped with delight because it's so gorgeous you've had to have it? Or you've bought something because it looked so fantastic on your friend but somehow it sits unworn in the wardrobe because it doesn't look quite right on you.

I know I've done it countless times. For me, it's usually when I'm trying to look feminine or when there's a big event coming up like a wedding or a party. The garment in question is usually something with a definite waist and a feminine feel to it. I ache to look like a real woman (think Marilyn Monroe), sexy and alluring - but I don't. I actually look more like the crocheted dolly Hyacinth Bucket (sorry Bouquet) would use to cover her toilet roll. As with everything, there is a good, scientific reason for this.

Think about Christmas and the time you spend wrapping all those presents. I don't know about you but I'm not too bad when the gift is a book or a box of some sort but as soon as I attempt to wrap something with curved edges I start having problems.

The same problem can also apply to "wrapping" our bodies. Trying to dress a curvy body in a stiff, starchy fabric is as difficult as wrapping a golf ball in an envelope. It won't fit properly unless lots of adjustments are made. Even the most expensive paper will not enhance the shape of the object. Furthermore, the package tends to look both bigger and thrown together, however hard you've tried.

Conversely, a straight, angular object like a ruler does not fit well inside a flimsy wrapping. The corners poke through and the wrapping easily slips.

I'm not suggesting any of us is completely rotund or as straight as a stick but all of us lean more towards one shape than the other. I often see curvier women wearing cotton shift dresses, usually with a round neck and no sleeves, thinking they will hide their bodies but, in actual fact, all they are doing is making themselves look bigger and less shapely.

I remember the surprise and delight of one of my clients with this type of figure, after we divested her of this type of garment. A gently flared skirt and a jacket with a nipped in waist made her look and feel like a siren. Her figure was back and it was terrific.

Looking at your body in an objective way and understanding your unique shape will determine how you can dress it in a way that will always look fantastic. Looking good and feeling great are inextricably linked. Understanding your body and being able to capitalise on the best bits will provide you with the means to create your own personal style. Neither contoured (round) or angular (straight) is the best option, as both can look terrific if you understand some of the style principles and use them accordingly.

Step 1: Take a good look in a full length mirror – preferably in your undies.

- Work from the shoulders and down to your waist area.

- Do your shoulders slope or are they straight?

- Are your upper arms and shoulders softly padded or are they quite bony?

- Is your waist defined with hips that flare or do you have no discernible waistline?

Turn to the side view:

- Is your bust larger than a D cup or smaller?

- Does the small of your back curve in or is it straight?

If you answered mainly yes to the first part of the questions then your upper body is contoured. If you answered mainly yes to the second part then it's angular.

Step 2: Let's look at your bottom half.

Turn to the front view:

- Do you have definite hips that curve or are they 'boyish'?

- Do you have a curve around the saddle bag area or are your legs straight?

Turn again to the side:

- Is your bottom rounded or flattish?

- Do you have a tum or do you have a flat abdomen?

If you answered yes to the first part of the question then your upper body is contoured. If you answered yes to the second part then it's angular.

It is possible to have a different bodyline for the upper and lower halves of your body and if this is the case, you must treat them differently. You may also have difficulty buying fitted dresses because of this.

The line of your body is really important because it determines not only the best shapes for your clothing but also the types of fabric, the cut, the patterns and the finishes that will really enhance the way you look.

In my case, the 50s film star look is designed to accommodate luscious curves, of which I have none. My attempt to look more 'feminine' revolved around emulating the success of a curvier woman to achieve this look rather than dressing to enhance my own angular uniqueness. I am able to look 'sexy' but not in this type of garment. As someone with a 'boyish' body, I am better creating femininity with accessories, a discreet frill, colour or makeup than full-blown burlesque.

Picture Dolly Parton trying to fit into a stiff cotton shirt. She may pull it of because of who she is, but for most of us, it doesn't work. You will look as though you are fighting with your clothes. They won't sit properly and you'll be constantly fiddling with them, so you'll appear ill at ease.

Here are my guidelines to help you dress your body so that you'll always look and feel fabulous.

THE SHAPE

If you have any curves at all, there needs to be a corresponding curve in the cut of the garment or you'll visually gain weight. If you have a waist, you need a waist in your jacket. A hollow back needs to be semi-fitted by use of darts or the extra fabric will hang and your great asset will be hidden. A curve in the hip needs trousers that also have a curve from the waist which is clearly visible when you hold them up on the hanger. If they are straight from waist to leg, guess what – they won't fit properly and they'll create draglines that pull, making you look like you've squeezed into clothes that are too small, or the waist will gape at the back.

If like me, you have few curves, don't pick clothes with full skirts and tiny waistbands or tops that obviously need a large bust to fill them. Work with your own silhouette to look the best you can.

FABRICS

Rounded bodies (contoured) look best in soft fabrics that drape and skim. The fabric should be able to move with you rather than constrict. It should enhance your curves rather than squash or flatten. If you are very muscular, go for semi taut as anything too floppy will not support your musculature. If it pulls across the chest, the thighs or the bum, don't buy it. If there are see-through gaps on a button-fastening shirt or dress, put it back.

Straighter (angular) bodies suit stiff, starchy fabrics. This applies to all items of clothing including jeans (Lycra is for contoured bodies and will quickly 'sag' on a straighter shape). A problem for you can be too much fabric on the hips or bust areas or the softness of the fabric making you look really 'hard' and sticklike.

PATTERNS

Patterns and designs look great if they reflect your overall bodyline. Stripes, checks and other geometric shapes enhance the lines of an angular body. Abstract patterns, curves, spots, paisley and florals suit a contoured shape. Everyone can wear plain fabrics, but be aware of texture as it can add bulk to a larger figure. It's best worn on a body where the top and bottom halves differ in their shape. Someone with an angular top and contoured bottom would look great in a cable knit sweater but someone who is contoured all over would look much larger. Shiny fabrics also have an enlarging affect while matt fabrics slim, so don't wear shine on a particular part of your body if you don't want anyone to notice it.

The cut of a garment is essential to make the most of your natural shape but the details often go unnoticed. These can make a huge difference between something that looks 'OK' and one that says 'wow'. Follow your overall silhouette guidelines and look for straight seams, sharp lapels, slash pockets and straight hems if you are angular. Rounded lapels, curved seams (or less structure if you're larger), rounded hems and pockets with flaps suit the curvier figure.

SIZE MATTERS

Please don't get fixated with the size label in your garments. There is no standardisation of sizing in the UK for female clothing. Even in the same store, you can find a size 10 may be bigger than a size 12. If the label upsets you – cut it out and throw it away. At the end of the day, a great fit is what really counts.

However, size does matter in a slightly different context. Fabric weight and patterns, accessories and heel height will look considerably better if the size you choose reflects that of your body. If not, you're in danger of looking eccentric, over-powering or lost.

Dame Edna Everage is not an icon you'd wish to emulate, but she does demonstrate the point. Everything she wears, from her over-sized specs, to the glittery costumes and the 'big' hair yell bad taste.

Look at the diagram below:

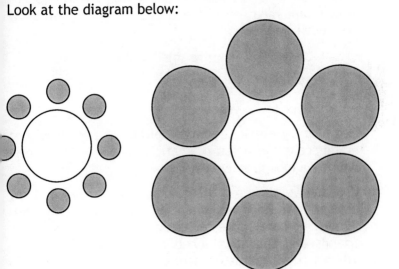

Which of the inner circles looks the smaller?

Actually the circles are the same size. The one surrounded by the larger circles only appears to be smaller because it is overshadowed by the larger ones.

If you wear clothes or patterns that are too large for you, you will appear swamped - not smaller, just lost. If you're larger than you'd like to be it's not an easy get out clause or an alternative to exercise or eating sensibly I'm afraid. Conversely, if you wear too small a scale, you will look much bigger. Can't believe many of us would want that!

You'll be pleased to know that scale is relative to bone structure and not to the amount of fat you carry. So ladies, when I ask you to find a tape measure, hopefully, you'll not have a heart attack.

This is not an exact science but it works well enough. Take a tape measure and measure around your wrist. If your wrist measures:

- Under 5½" - you're small scale
- 5½ - 6½" - medium
- Over 6½" - grand

Don't worry about the words either. A person with a grand scale can be so dramatic in the way they dress and it's a look I really envy.

I've always hankered after what I can't have and my clothes have been no exception (in the past anyway). Flimsy, romantic dresses seemed to really suit my friends and they all looked fantastic wearing them. When I tried – disaster struck. I looked like a man in drag – seriously. The materials that I chose to create femininity were too lightweight for my medium scale. Bones I didn't even know I had poked through the fabric, the straps kept falling down my shoulders, my bust became non-existent (this _is_ bad news) and I looked, and felt, really uncomfortable. Not how you want to feel when attending an important event. In addition, the fabric of my floaty outfit didn't suit my angular body as there is no stiffness in its mix. The only way I could have 'rescued' it would have been to wear something more structured in a thicker material underneath. Probably better to choose something more flattering in the first place.

To get an idea of scale worn badly, imagine a lady with a fuller figure spilling over the edge of her small, kitten heels or a tiny, petite one in huge platform shoes. Get the idea?

So here are guidelines for you to think about:

Fabric weights should be worn according to your own body's scale. So light-weight for small scale, medium for medium scale and slightly heavier weight for grand scale.

Patterns should also reflect your bodyline, so a small floral pattern would look great on a small scale, contoured woman.

Accessories. A small, floppy handbag will look fantastic on a small scale contoured woman but a large square tote will completely dwarf her.

Shoes should have a heel and sole size corresponding to scale. Dainty shoes do not suit grand scale women,

If you are a mixture of extremes, for example 6'1", size 8-10 with small wrists and ankles or 4'11", size 18 plus with large bones, opt always for medium scale.

The size of a pattern can also affect the visual weight of a fabric (as opposed to the physical weight). A light-weight chiffon printed with large scale flowers in deep or bright multi colours will look heavier on the wearer than a pastel coloured chiffon with a small pattern or no design.

I remember one of my wardrobe-weeding sessions with a client who had a small to medium frame. She showed me her brand new coat, patterned with very large roses over the entire garment. I was *very* keen to let it go, she was adamant it was staying. In the end, I donned the coat myself and asked her for her opinion. She burst out laughing. I looked like a garden trellis! We had no problem disposing of it after that. The coat would have looked fantastic on someone with a larger scale so choose your patterns with care.

The texture of a fabric is also important. As I said before, a shiny fabric will make you look larger than a matt one. Just think of a man with a beer belly in a shiny football shirt and you'll know what I mean. So use matt fabrics if you don't want to attract attention to a certain part of your body. This also applies to light and dark colours. A dark colour will make you look slimmer than a lighter one. So beware of wearing light, shiny fabrics on areas that you're not comfortable showing off.

On the whole a textured garment will create a softer outline than one with sharp tailoring. If you have an angular body, you are better off steering clear of loose, nubby type fabrics. Stick to fabrics that are tightly woven like gabardine or twill. If you are very curvy, texture can add bulk to your frame, so choose fabrics that fall in soft folds such as jersey, wool crepe and wool/silk blends.

My scale is

....

Fabric weight is

....

Patterns are

....

....

....

....

Accessories

....

....

....

....

....

Drama can be created by up-scaling. A large piece of jewellery, a higher heel, a huge belt buckle or a bolder pattern can all get you noticed. Just choose ONE area only or you'll end up looking like Dame Edna. We want drama not pantomime.

To be truly authentic in the way you dress, you will need to 'imitate' your features within your clothing as it creates a kind of rhythm, which is often hard to put your finger on but always looks amazing. If you have freckled skin, for instance, you will look great in a textured, multi-coloured scarf. If you have thick hair, opt for thickness in one of your fabrics. If you have smooth skin, you'll look better in smooth, satiny materials. Repeat your eye colour in your garments or your accessories for that added 'je ne sais quoi'.

As we get older, our hair turns greyer and our lines become more pronounced. This means we can open up to new possibilities in our clothing. The once smooth fabrics might now give way to textured or patterned. Grey hair could look absolutely fabulous matched with a long grey evening dress and silver accessories. The important thing is to make changes that reflect the change in you.

A word about quality. In the past, it was always the unwritten rule that you should buy the best quality fabrics you could afford when purchasing your clothes. These days, it seems that people are in two camps: those who buy designer labels and bespoke tailoring and those who prefer the 'throw away' culture of cheaper items. With top names designing for High Street stores you can achieve a stylish look at a great price. Even the well known celebs pair luxury designer garments with those from chain stores on the High Street. The let down is always with the accessories. Unless you're looking for a 'fun' look, choose accessories that are classic and show quality and good taste. At important meetings, for instance, you can bet money on the fact that your shoes, bag, watch and jewellery will be noticed.

Remember, fit is everything. You can spend thousands of pounds on designer labels but if they don't fit you properly, don't enhance your silhouette or aren't appropriate for your lifestyle, they are destined for the charity shop before you've even got them home. With the cheaper end of the market, fit is even more important because the quality of the fabrics is less forgiving. These days I tend to invest in key pieces like a great jacket, rather then three or four from the High Street. Cheaper items satisfy my 'fashionista' side, so I'll wear them to death all season and then discard. It pays to be very discerning with really fashionable items as they can look ridiculous on our age group. I'm afraid floral smocks just didn't do it for me last year so I had to adopt a more classic approach. As a rule my basic guideline is 80% classic and 20% trend, though this may depend on your style preferences – see 'The Real Deal' chapter for more information on why you buy what you do.

I always spend money on great handbags, as these are my real, true passion. Each one makes a statement; so much so, I get complete strangers stopping to admire them in the street. Whenever I put a beautiful bag on my shoulder I feel a great sense of joy. It's so easy to ring the changes to basic colours and clothing by swapping your bag and shoes, especially as there are some really unusual colours and designs out there at the moment.

If you can't decide whether a garment or an accessory is really worth what you're paying for it, ask yourself "Does it have the wow factor?" If it doesn't then walk away, because you're bound to find something you'd rather have just around the corner. If you're still thinking (dreaming) about it days later, then go back and revisit your decision. Odds are you'll probably have forgotten about it but if you haven't, perhaps it was meant to be. Consider whether your new purchase will complement your existing wardrobe and will it actually get worn. Spending thousands on a dress you'll wear once may be slightly over the top unless the occasion really does warrant that type of investment.

When you are trying on clothes in a shop, walk around in the changing rooms, sit down and see what happens. Has the garment creased? Does it restrict you in any way? Is it comfortable as well as flattering? Do you *love* it? You understand your shape and scale so work with what you've got and don't fight against it.

WORDS OF WISDOM

✓ Love what you buy only if it loves you back.

✓ If you can't find anything suitable for a particular occasion, don't panic buy. Work with what you already own and change the way it looks using accessories.

✓ Never wear matching accessories and that includes jewellery sets – it's very dating.

✓ Beware of wearing anything too trendy from top to toe.

Nobody's Perfect
(How To Look Like A Model)

"My legs aren't so beautiful. I just know what to do with them."

MARLENE DIETRICH

Whether or not we spend money on quality clothing, most of us no longer look like the models and celebrities we see in magazines. I can't airbrush you, but I can show you how to cheat so you'll certainly look more model-like than you did before.

Apart from being beautiful, models have something else - Perfect Proportions:

- shoulders wider than hips
- long waist
- long legs

As long as we can create the illusion of having these proportions in our own bodies, we too can look like we belong on the catwalk.

The first thing to do is to understand your own proportions. When we measure proportion we are looking at the ratio of one part of the body to another in order to create balance.

First of all, let's look at your legs versus your body. By the way, if you are very tall this does not automatically mean you have long legs proportionally speaking. You'll always have a longer measurement than someone of average size but you may still have short legs. This is quite difficult to do on your own so you might need a partner to help.

Sit bolt upright against a wall making sure your back is straight and your bottom is touching the skirting board, creating a 90 degree angle. Mark where the top of your head touches the wall. Stand up and measure the distance. Now measure your own full height. If the distance on the wall is more than half your height, you are long bodied. If it's shorter, you are long legged. If the distances are equal, you have perfect proportions but follow the guidelines for short legs just to make you look even more fabulous.

Generally speaking, if you are long bodied you will have short legs and vice versa. Naturally large breasted women tend to be short bodied and long legged. Lucky you – large boobs and long legs. Those of us with long bodies often have flat tummies, no bust and a low bottom with saddlebags – but not always.

Now check your hips, as we want to make them as small as possible: Stand in front of a mirror and check whether the edges of your shoulders are wider or narrower than your hips at the widest point. If unsure, hold the edge of a ribbon against your outer shoulder and let it drop towards your hips. If it misses, then you have wider shoulders. If it touches, you have wider or the same size hips.

My proportions are

1. Legs/body ....

2. Shoulders/hips ....

I am one of those people who at 5'4" has a very long body and really short legs. Delegates at my workshops are amazed when I tell them as I've managed to hide it extremely well. They believe I am taller than my actual height and have legs that go on forever. I use my knowledge to change what I haven't got naturally into something I'd love to have. Who cares if it's cheating?

Here's how it can work for you:

SHORT LEGS/LONG BODY

The general principle here is short - shorter length jackets, shorter length tops and shorter length skirts. The longest jackets to suit you will just cover the cheeks of your bottom. Any longer and your legs will shorten. Skirt and coat hems should sit around knee length.

✓ Avoid turn ups on trousers as the horizontal line will shorten the leg. And definitely avoid any trousers with tapered legs. Make sure they are long enough. They should touch where your toes crease. If you are petite, you can afford to have trousers trailing on the ground.

✓ Boot cut is very flattering for shorter legs.

✓ Vertical stripes or a centre crease give the illusion of length.

✓ Shorter skirts (knee length) are more flattering than long ones. Wear with knee high boots that touch the hem of the skirt or co-ordinating tights. Any gap will shorten the leg. Asymmetric hems are also a good idea.

✓ Pointed toe shoes will lengthen, rounded will shorten, as will any horizontal bars in the design. Avoid ankle straps at all costs, especially if calves are thick. Try flip-flop V designs rather than sliders in the summer.

✓ Heels make legs look longer as do shoes with platform soles.

✓ Jackets should be no longer than bum length. Shorter jackets look good as long as you have no challenges round the hip or tum area.

✓ Belts should match bottoms rather than tops.

✓ A ¾ length sleeve or a sleeve pushed up will lengthen the leg optically.

LONG LEGS / SHORT WAIST

The general principle here is long - longer jackets, longer tops and longer skirts. A flattering jacket length would probably just cover the cheeks of your bottom. If you wear a shorter jacket, your waist will also shorten and you will look out of proportion. Unless it's a pencil skirt, most skirt and coat hems look better worn long, between calf and ankle, with the shortest at knee level.

✓ Avoid any horizontal lines on your top half as they will widen and make you look fatter. Vertical lines will slim.

✓ Drop-waisted or hipster trousers give length to your upper body.

✓ Single-breasted jackets and cardigans flatter whilst double breasted will give the illusion of width. Keep your jacket open and wear a column of the same colour underneath if you want to appear slimmer.

✓ Empire line dresses and tops will give the illusion of length in the torso, as will tops with an asymmetric hemline.

✓ Try trousers and skirts without waistbands.

✓ If you do wear a belt, match it to your top half not the bottom.

✓ Wear shirts and tops worn out rather than tucked in.

✓ Longer skirts and jacket lengths look good but be careful of where the hemlines stop. If they cut across a problem area such as very wide hips or calves, you will gain visual weight.

✓ You can wear flat shoes but not at the expense of frumpiness. Podiatrists now agree that a ½" heel is better for your feet than none at all.

NARROW SHOULDERS

✓ Wide lapels and shirt collars give the illusion of width.

✓ Avoid halter necks as all eyes will be on your boobs. Also avoid raglan, three quarter or sleeveless garments.

✓ Trench coats with detail on the shoulder can work well if you're not too busty.

✓ Sleeves such as capped, petal, dolman or ruched will automatically widen the shoulderline.

✓ Off-the-shoulder styles look good or try wrapping a scarf or pashmina round your shoulders.

✓ Shoulder pads (as long as they are a discreet part of your tailoring) can provide balance with the hips.

✓ Avoid excessive pleating or bulk around the hips as this will also make your shoulders look out of proportion.

✓ The use of colour can also help distract attention away from the shoulders. Wear darker colours on your bottom half to make the hips look smaller and your shoulders wider. Bright or light colours in shiny fabrics will attract attention and your shoulders will appear larger while dark colours in a matt fabric will deflect and narrow.

✓ For the best placement of zips and seams in skirts and trousers, take a look at your waist from the side view. If it's narrower than the front view, wear zips and seams in the centre front of your garment. If your waist is pretty much the same size all round, move the zip/seam to the side. It gives the illusion of a slimmer profile.

FIGURE CHALLENGES

I know from experience, my own and my clients', that we often have a problem with a certain area of our body. So much so, that we often fixate on it - even though other people rarely notice or cannot understand what we're worried about. If it's real for you, it won't make much difference what others say, it will still cause you concern.

I have a very low-slung bum due to my very long back. From the front I look OK but from the back I always feel my bum is drooping further and further towards my knees. You may not notice this but I do – and that's what counts.

I've now developed a look that completely hides my bum, still gives me a great outline and always looks stylish. A fitted jacket, with a knee length hem, can be worn over jeans, trousers and a skirt. As long as I team it with heels, so I remain in proportion, you cannot tell where my bum is and the rest of my body looks great.

This type of jacket also works well to disguise saddlebags. I have also started to wear longer sweaters as my tummy is starting to expand now I'm menopausal. Knitwear, which I've always worn with a waist length hem, can ride up making me feel exposed round my middle. As long as I stick to my longer trousers and add a heel, this is perfectly OK for my proportions.

What would never work is a longer jumper worn with flat shoes and/or tapered trousers like skinny jeans for instance. I could never (ever) leave the house wearing those. You couldn't believe how awful that particular combination would look.

If you have no problems with any part of your body, you can skip the rest of this chapter and move onto the next one. If, like me, gravity is taking its toll – keep reading.

FULL BUST

✓ Women with large boobs often have a short neck. An opening at the neck, such as a V-neck or a scoop, will break up the area. Try open neck shirts (the stand up collar will flatter the face), or a crossover V sweater. A closed neckline, for instance a polo neck or mandarin collar, will make the bust appear larger.

✓ A full bust means a contoured outline, so stick to curved lines on top. Avoid details and prints that draw focus to the breasts, especially horizontal stripes or pockets.

✓ The correct bra is essential. It can take pounds off you. Don't wear lacy bras with t-shirts or close fitting fabrics.

✓ Dark colours in a matt fabric will draw attention from the bust area. Bright colours and shiny fabrics attract attention to it.

✓ Longer line jackets, with single-breasted fastenings and long sleeves look great on large busts. Try wearing a scarf draped round the neck and falling over the chest area to create length.

✓ Ruching is great as you can't tell what is you and what is fabric, so this design feature hides a multitude of sins.

✓ Avoid halter neck tops, especially with unsupported boobs, or tops with sleeves ending at the bust line.

SMALL BUST

✓ Padded bras and "chicken fillets" are a must if you want to look like you have a cleavage. Aim for a smooth finish under clingier fabrics. Most stores sell seamless t-shirt bras which do the job well.

✓ Wearing lots of thin layers can add bulk to the chest area without making you look fat.

✓ Ruching is good as you can't tell between bust size and fabric.

✓ Pockets, stripes and patterns placed on the bustline enhance the chest.

✓ Short sleeves ending at the bust line create a horizontal line creating width.

✓ Off-the-shoulder, halter necks, patterns and textures look great on a smaller chest.

✓ Light colours in shiny fabrics attract attention.

✓ Avoid necklines that are too low, and going bra-less.

A TUM

✓ To skim is to slim so dress to divert attention away from your mid section.

✓ Single-breasted jackets and coats will lengthen and slim the body, especially if they are longer length.

✓ Wear the same colour on upper and lower body.

✓ Try dresses and tops with an empire line or no visible waistline.

✓ Avoid belts round the waist or tops tucked in.

LARGE HIPS

✓ The focus needs to be drawn away from the bum and hips.

✓ Wear long jackets that don't cut across the hip line or your widest point.

✓ Dark colours on the bottom and lighter colours on your upper body will draw the attention away from your lower half.

✓ Jewellery and scarves worn higher on the body are good diversionary tactics.

✓ Boot cut trousers/jeans, trousers without waistbands, and drapey fabrics that don't cling are a wise choice.

✓ Avoid too much detail around the waist such as belt loops or pleating.

FLABBY UPPER ARMS

Unfortunately, this is something that comes to all of us, despite how many tricep dips we do at the gym. My arms look great when I'm flexing my muscles but when I wave, suddenly the whole of my upper arm wobbles. So unless you are absolutely sure your arm is well defined and strong, you may want to cover up. A pashmina casually draped around the arms is sexy for eveningwear and ¾ sleeves are very flattering if you have short legs.

SUN-DAMAGED DÉCOLLETAGE AND NECK

Try not to use this area as a main focus if your skin is crepey, marked or wrinkled. Frame your face with open collars, use a scarf or polo neck to cover and wear flattering colours against your face to draw the eye upwards. A full necklace that covers the area will work as well but beware of very bright metal jewellery as it will exacerbate the damage.

If you do wear a scarf wrapped round your neck and throat, roll up your sleeves so that you aren't completely covered and some flesh is on show, otherwise you'll look unbalanced.

SAGGY KNEES

I tend to wear trousers or thick tights to cover mine but you can also lower your skirt hemlines if you like a more feminine look. Don't buy shiny tights as this will make your legs look bigger.

MOTTLED HANDS

Thank goodness gloves have made a comeback, though not practical in summer I know. Wear them whenever you can. I have ¾ length ones which I wear with shorter sleeved jackets and they are very glam. If you don't like your hands, avoid excess jewellery as it will attract attention. I'm not overly keen on more than one ring on each hand anyway as it looks gaudy, so stick to the less-is-more philosophy.

PETITE

If you're under 5'2" you will probably need to find a specialist range of clothing that will cater for your proportions. Many stores stock petite ranges these days but beware of covering too much of your body. Long skirts and long sleeves often 'drown' a smaller lady. Sleeves can look better worn at ¾ length and skirts with a knee length hem.

Karen Gillam designs clothes specifically for women up to 5'3" and has kindly given me her top tips to pass on:

- ✓ Keep **PROPORTIONS** high with empire lines, short jackets and tops whilst keeping accessories and patterns on a smaller scale.

- ✓ **EMPHASISE** the waist with well-shaped garments avoiding loose, ill fitting, wide or bulky clothes.

- ✓ **TONE** or link colours from top to toe.

- ✓ **INVESTMENT** dressing is important.

- ✓ Appear **TALLER** and slimmer with vertical style lines.

- ✓ Emphasise **ELEGANT** ankles with low cut shoes, no ankle straps.

For more information contact Karen Gillam at Karen Gillam Petite Collection, Dress Code UK Ltd, 0845 0035049, *www.karengillam.co.uk*

TALL

Despite most models being very tall, this can be tricky. Many trousers are cut too short and sleeves often end high above the wrist causing a dangling hand. I've found that Zara is very good if you are around the 6' mark.

For longer lengths, try Long Tall Sally (*www.longtallsally.com*) or TallGirls (*www.tallgirls.co.uk*) and bear in mind that M&S now do an extra long trouser.

LARGER

I'm not always a big fan of the High Street as I feel that they often take a size 10 model and just incrementally increase the size of the garment rather than taking into account the differing proportions of a larger build. Try *www.box2.co.uk* sizes 14-30 for clothes which are European in origin and a bit different, or the online store Simply Be (*www.simplybe.co.uk*).

If all else fails, move the focus upwards towards your face or downwards towards your feet by adding colour or a bold accessory.

When my face looks pretty much like a bloodhound, I get out my bright red, killer shoes. Never fails. The attention always moves to my feet. Why? You'll need to read the chapter on colour – 'It's Not All Black and White'.

WORDS OF WISDOM

✓ Follow the guidelines above but adapt to camouflage any areas of concern.

✓ When trying on skirts, move the skirt upwards so the hem is higher by an inch or so. Does it look better or would the skirt look better with a longer hem? Skirts with hemlines worn touching the crease at the back of the knee are very youthful.

✓ Do the same with your jacket. Short jackets worn with trousers can make the bottom look big from the rear view or highlight a long rise. Overly long jackets can shorten the legs dramatically. As jackets are difficult to alter, don't buy unless the length is right.

✓ Check your trousers are long enough. Better to be too long than too short.

✓ Learn how to disguise any problem areas and then really focus on your assets and make them a key feature.

✓ Show flesh discreetly as it will add mystery and allure.

✓ If it's hot, use layers of thinner fabrics to stay cool and avoid over exposure.

Winter Wonderland

"My coat and I are comfortable together. I only feel its presence because it keeps me warm."

VICTOR HUGO

I for one am delighted when summer is over and the crisp smell of autumn is upon us. Don't get me wrong, I love the heat and I appreciate that everything looks better when the sun is out. My problem is summer clothes, or specifically my wearing them.

I'm sure I never had this problem before the age of 40, but somehow summers now seem to take so much effort when it comes to deciding what to wear.

I reckon women are split into two camps: those who love the winter and those who prefer the sun. If you absolutely love hot weather and the clothes you can wear, you have my permission to skip the rest of this chapter. If like me, you have a preference for wrapping up in woolly knits, boots and a scarf, please read on.

As I've aged, baring my legs to the world just doesn't have the same appeal. Saggy knees and varicose veins don't look attractive when they are lily white and we all know that excessive sun bathing is a no-no – if only someone had told me earlier. In years past, I burned like a sausage on a spit, resplendent in an olive oil coating just so I could have skin the colour of old mahogany furniture. These days, unprotected feet result in massive blisters (I need my socks), and hobbling along in high-heeled sandals doesn't have the same effect when your toes are swollen like cocktail sausages.

There is also the dilemma of depilation. We all know waxing is better for long term results, but who wants to show off hairy pins in the interim? Wobbly upper arms are another source of discomfort and we realise too late that we should have visited the gym at least a few times a week before now. The alternative of long sleeves isn't a pleasant option for us 'older' women, as we are more likely to sweat, sorry 'glow'.

What about the workplace? In the US, legs without hose is considered a major faux pas and women who dare to bare are considered to be the bottom of the heap in terms of promotional prospects. Sandals, toe cleavage and skirts worn above knee level are considered 'tarty' so no respite there either. Do we continue to sweat away in our corporate suits and pray for fierce, air conditioning in our offices and cars? Looking at some office workers, I suspect not.

How envious I am of those of you who look great in skimpy tops, flip flops and floaty skirts. You seem to have radiance and an ease that I can never match at this heat-soaked time of the year. Summer people often tend towards the natural and have no need for protective makeup to look fresh and dewy. Compare that with us winter types who can't move without our face on and consider the beach a nightmare unless waterproof foundation and lippy are in place.

So winter ladies, what can we do, apart from hibernating or holidaying at the North Pole? Here are some tips for summer dressing without baring all:

✓ Choose loose cut, long linen trousers instead of shorts. Make sure, if they have a drawstring fastening, that they are not bulky round the waist.

✓ Pashminas and open knit shrugs are great for hiding upper arms.

✓ ¾ length sleeves look better than those that finish at bust level – leave them for the men to wear.

✓ If you wear a skirt, choose ankle length or an asymmetric hemline.

✓ A light coloured, cotton shirt, teamed with a pair of jeans can look really 'on trend' and timeless too.

✓ Choose natural fibres so your body can breathe. Layering them means you can look stylish and stay cool.

✓ Wedge shoes give more stability to the foot than high heeled sandals without compromising on elegance or leg length.

✓ Draw attention towards the face with fabulous jewellery and/or sunglasses.

✓ Fake tans are now really good, don't streak and are devoid of that awful smell they used to have. Spray tans only take a few minutes and the results can be very natural. Beware though if you have very white, porcelain-like skin as it might look too yellow and you'll look ill instead of healthy.

✓ Wear gorgeous hats to keep your face in the shade, preventing sunspots and other age giveaways at the same time.

WORDS OF WISDOM

✓ Whether you are a winter or a summer type, don't forget to wear adequate sunscreen.

✓ Sitting outside for fifteen minutes every day can really help you increase your Vitamin D levels. Try not to stay out at mid-day as it's too hot.

Here Comes The Sun

"People shop for a bathing suit with more care than they do for a husband or wife. The rules are the same. Look for something you'll feel comfortable wearing. Allow for room to grow."

ERMA BOMBECK

Summer is no longer just confined to a couple of months a year. With holidays abroad costing so little these days, we can spend as much time in the sun as our bank accounts allow. How do you feel about exposing your flesh to the scrutiny of other holidaymakers? If the answer is "I hate it", then take heed of the following advice. Swimwear exists to suit all shapes and sizes. It's just a question of knowing what will make you look even more gorgeous than you already are.

Here are my tips to help enhance your best features and disguise those that you don't like as much.

LARGE HIPS

✓ If you have large hips or saddlebags along with a smallish bust, opt for a two-piece rather than a swimsuit.

✓ Small bikini bottoms, especially those with string ties at the side, will elongate legs.

✓ Halter necks and ruched tops will create a more balanced bustline.

✓ Bikini bottoms with a V cut waistband will also work.

✓ Bandeau tops look great if they are cinched in the middle rather than going straight across the chest area.

✓ Many bikinis have different patterns/colours top and bottom so make the most of the new trend. Dark colours on your bottom half will make it look slimmer, whilst a bright or light colour top will divert attention away from the hip area.

✓ If you really don't feel comfortable in a bikini, buy a one piece with high cut legs or try a tankini with a smaller bottom.

✓ If you have a large bum, don't choose high-waisted bottoms or those that completely cover all of your cheeks. You will look matronly and frumpy and your backside will grow at least two sizes.

✓ A sarong wrapped loosely round the waist and a large sunhat to balance, completes the look. Carry a bright patterned beach bag over your shoulder to also divert attention away from your hips and balance out your body.

LARGE TUM

✓ A one-piece swimsuit is the best bet. If you can find one with ruching down the centre, even better, as the wrinkles disguise any flesh in the folds of the fabric.

✓ Depending on your overall size, you can use a pattern to detract the eye from the offending area.

✓ If you have large boobs, you will need a swimsuit that has a lowish neck or your bust can appear 'shelf-like' and even more obvious.

✓ A swimsuit with a medium high cut leg will make the most of longer legs and detract attention away from your middle.

✓ To cover up, try a V-neck kaftan and a big pair of sunspecs.

LARGE BOOBS

✓ Avoid halter or high necklines as they will make your bust look enormous.

✓ Tops should have support under the bust but make sure it is stylish. You don't want to look like a grandma.

✓ A keyhole top can be surprisingly effective, and it's also very glamorous.

✓ A sarong tied around the waist is your best cover up option. If you tie it higher on the body or with a halter twist around the neck, it will attract attention to your bust.

ANGULAR

✓ A halter neck top will widen shoulders and boobs will appear to be larger.

✓ If you are long bodied, try a tankini, as it may feel more comfortable. You can wear athletic looking swimwear, so try racing backs.

✓ Beware of triangle tops, as they can flatten your breasts if not padded. Bandeau tops, in a textured or detailed fabric can flatter and add inches, as can strategically placed 'chicken fillets'.

✓ If you want to look curvier, opt for a swimsuit with keyholes cut out of the sides. Boy shorts can work, if you have long legs. If your legs are short, avoid at all costs as you'll look stumpy.

✓ A pair of linen drawstring trousers looks great on this shape. Try a baseball cap, a bandanna or a small bucket hat as your finishing accessory. Alternatively, try a sarong tied around the bust.

CURVY

✓ Keep it simple. Block colours look best as they elongate your frame. Choose underwired bra tops, whether in a bikini or a swimsuit, as droopy boobs are not a good look to have. A belted one-piece looks great if you have a tiny waist and you want to create an hour glass figure.

✓ A sarong, a large hat and huge sunspecs will give you film star appeal. Avoid a kaftan as it will hide your curves and make you appear larger.

✓ For those of you who are drama queens, bring out your film star element. Buy some super sunglasses, add a cocktail (or two) and act as if you are the belle of the beach. Relax in the knowledge that you look terrific.

WORDS OF WISDOM

✓ Think about your scale and your complexion. Too large a pattern on a petite frame can swamp and too small on a large frame can add pounds. Black can be slimming, on the right colouring. If you are naturally fair-haired, and don't tan well, black may be overpowering. Try brown or blue instead.

✓ Size and fit is critical. Never purchase swimwear if you have to keep adjusting the legs or if it's too short in the body. Persevere. The perfect garment awaits you.

✓ Shoes with a wedge or thick sole, coupled with a V frontage such as a flip-flop, will lengthen the legs. Sliders, or any sandal with a horizontal bar, will shorten.

✓ Unless you have a bright complexion (see the chapter 'It's Not All Black and White'), steer clear of very bright or garish colours until you have your tan. Stick to muted, neutral tones so you don't look washed out.

✓ A fake tan can increase your well-being and make you look slimmer.

✓ Your hair can suffer with too much heat, so buy a conditioner with in built sunscreen, a heavy-duty hair mask to keep it looking healthy, or sport a great hat.

✓ Unless you have the perfect body, cover up with a beautiful sarong, flattering linen trousers or a large, flowing shirt when walking around. Too much flesh on display can be very off putting.

True Colours (It's Not All Black And White)

"Pink is not a colour, it's a state of mind."

ANON

If I had a pound for every woman I saw wearing black on a regular basis, I'd be a millionaire by now. As we get older, and often larger, we look to black as our safe option. We think it makes us look smaller and more sophisticated. In fact 76% of women's clothes sold in UK annually are black. If you are one of the many women that don't really suit black, you may be making yourself look tired and drawn instead of slim and chic.

Hundreds of years ago, man did not have names for all the colours we have today. Modern technology has produced a myriad of new shades for us to delight in. One way of labelling that has been with us from the start is that of a warm shade (yellow based) and a cool one (blue based). They also were aware of terms such as dark and light, bright and soft. These characteristics are what we base our colour analysis on today. By using specific coloured drapes, we can pick out colours which share the same characteristics as the complexion, thus making you look wonderful when you wear them.

It's quite difficult to write successfully about which colours suit you the most. It is far better to have a consultation with a professional if you want to get it absolutely right. The Federation of Image Consultants provides a list of local consultants on their website *www.tfic.org.uk*.

I have defined particular groups below to help you but you may belong to one or more of them depending on your own personal make-up. Use them as a guideline to ascertain what will work best.

Clients who wear their most flattering colours have reported that they have been told how marvellous they look even when suffering from a hangover. If you want a day off work, just wear colours that don't suit you near your face and you'll soon be speeding homewards.

UNDERSTANDING YOUR CHARACTERISTICS

Generally speaking if you are dark haired, dark eyed with a dark skin or one that tans easily, you will wear dark colours well.

Conversely, if you are fair-haired, with a paler skin and eye colour, you will better suit lighter colours.

If you have red hair and freckles, or olive skin and green eyes, you will have a warm complexion so yellow-based colours will best suit you.

If you have a pink tone to your skin, blue eyes with ash-blonde or grey hair you'll have a cool complexion and blue-based colours will look great on you.

If you have a high contrast between hair and skin (black hair and very pale skin) or your eyes are very bright, you wear bright colours well.

If there is little contrast between hair, eyes and skin you are muted and suit softer colours.

There are two main systems used in colour analysis: directional, which determines characteristics that are most visible in the complexion and their order of significance; and seasonal, which specifies three characteristics which are grouped together and labelled as their corresponding part of the year. The latter is probably the most well known so I've used it in this book to explain the concept further, but neither system is better than the other – just slightly different. Both have been taken from The Munsell System of defining colour using the characteristics of undertone (hue), clarity (chroma) and depth (value). Hairdressers are familiar with the same system as it's used to code dyes and tints.

As with real life, there are four main types, or 'seasons', which I've detailed as follows:

WINTER Dark, Cool & Bright	AUTUMN Dark, Muted & Warm	SUMMER Light, Cool & Muted	SPRING Light, Bright & Warm
rk or grey ir	Golden blonde, auburn or brown hair	Light to medium ash blonde, mousy or cool light red hair	Golden blonde or warm light brunette/ red hair
ight blue, zel, brown black eyes	Soft shades of green, hazel or brown eyes	Pale blue, grey, green or hazel eyes	Bright shades of blue, green, hazel and brown
in can be r to very rk. It may ve a high ntrast to the ir	Skin tone is soft, similar to eye colour with no real contrast and will have a sun kissed look or freckles	Blue under-tones to the skin show in a pinkiness which can be fair or medium	Yellow undertones show as a sun kissed look on the skin, which will be fair.
ok of high ntrast or ength	Look of warmth or richness	Look of delicateness or, English rose	Look of lightness, and brightness

If you're unsure which box you fit into, use the guidelines for your dominant characteristic instead – if you know you are very dark, stick mainly to darker colours and accent with others.

If you do fit into a type shown above, it may be helpful to think about the colours you will find during each of the seasons, as these will be the ones that best suit you:

Winter: Bold, dramatic landscapes, with white snow, black trees shed of their leafage, grey skies, deep red berries. This palette includes the bright, deep primary colours, except yellow, and the icy tones of very pale blue, green, pink, violet and white. You can wear black and charcoal well and look fantastic in blocks of contrasting colours.

Autumn: Trees with leaves of all shades of gold, orange, green, yellow, red and brown give a good insight into the colours which suit this complexion. They are soft shades and not bright. Cream is a better choice than white. You will look better in chocolate brown or navy as your neutrals. Olive green looks especially good. Blend your colours together, for instance three shades of olive, rather than wearing obvious contrasts.

Summer: Soft shades of pink, lavender, blue and lemon. All pastels look good on this complexion. Imagine the sun has faded the colours of the flowers in bloom so they are no longer bright but have muted tones. Off-white is more suitable than a bright white. You will suit grey and a soft navy more than black for your basic neutrals. Like autumn, you wear blends of colours better than contrast.

Spring: Flowers are emerging such as daffodils, and crocuses. Bright shades that have a yellowish tinge but are light rather than dark. Corals, light green and turquoise fit nicely into this palette. Ivory is a better choice than white, which is too cool. You will look good in pale linen colours, beige or brown, rather than black. Wear a bright, vivid colour near the face to enliven the outfit or you could look jaded. Choosing your eye colour will work especially well.

Remember that these guidelines apply to colours worn around your face. If you love a colour and you know it doesn't suit you, wear it somewhere else. This is why I love my bags. I have every colour going. Some cost a fortune, others did not, but they all do a great job of allowing me to wear whatever colour fits my mood. My basic wardrobe revolves mainly around grey, which could be very dull on its own, especially for a vibrant personality like mine. Jewellery, shoes, a watch, a hair ornament or a belt can all pick up aspects of a colour that may be overwhelming if worn head to toe. A lipstick, a coloured mascara or unusual eyeliner will have the same effect.

Don't shy away from patterned or multi-coloured garments. As long as the overall colours suit you, a splash of another shade will not hurt. If the pattern is small or it's a textured garment, the colours may blend together so that from a distance it appears as a single colour.

It is important that you take your personality into account when you wear your colours. If you are shy, bright colours can propel you into an unwelcome limelight. We see bright colours first, due to their longer wavelengths, so try muted shades instead.

If you are bright, bold or dynamic you will probably look best in blocks of colour e.g. black trousers and white top. If you are softer or more gentle, try wearing the same colour in different values e.g. pale olive top with darker olive skirt and brown belt.

Remember that skin and hair fade as we age. You may feel overwhelmed by some colours that you'd have happily worn 20 years ago. I've certainly 'muted' my own look (especially lipstick colour) and I know I look younger as a result. You can sometimes go a little warmer if you are 'medium' colouring with no extremes or on the borderline of warm/cool as it can help you look younger but experiment (be curious) and gauge reactions before changing everything overnight.

Read the chapter on 'Fashion Feng Shui®' for more information on dressing your essence.

HAIR SPLITTING

Be wary of hairdressers and makeup advisors who don't understand the difference between cool and warm. The current trend is for us to be 'warmed up'. Cosmetic counters offer bronzing powers and fake tans to turn us into golden beauties, especially now sunbathing is strictly off limits. Hairdressers often promote gold or copper highlights to provide a warm glow around our face.

But being 'warmed up' doesn't actually suit all of us, especially as our colouring fades as we get older. In fact we can be in danger of looking jaundiced or sallow if we wear colours that are too yellow for our natural complexion. This can apply to fake tans too. Although safer than the lying in the sun, the golden look may not suit a naturally pale, cool skin. If you fall into this category, be brave and show off your natural pallor. It works for Nigella and Madonna. I'm not so sure it looks great on me, but I know I don't want skin cancer so I'm getting used to it (and being curious about the results).

If you have a cool skin tone, then look at shades of plum hair colour rather than auburn, ash-blonde or a mix of blond highlights rather than gold. If you have naturally fair hair, keep it fair and don't be tempted to go darker. Unfortunately, pigment does fade as we get older. So if your hair was naturally jet black (or very dark) it probably isn't now. Dying it back to its original shade will do you no favours. It will look harsh and artificial and you will look older and 'dated'. Opt for a colour about two shades lighter than your original to stay youthful. Highlights can add a natural movement and shine to your hair and are a safer alternative than an all-over colour. If you are grey, make the most of it by choosing a style that really shows off your crowning glory or soften slightly with some highlights.

For years I was a golden blonde. I never felt it was quite right but the hairdresser said it suited me and I went along with it. I applied stacks of makeup, bronzers and a really dark lipstick to balance out my look. Now I realise my instinct was correct. Enter a striking silver blonde. As this suits my colouring and my personality, I need less makeup, my eyes are brighter, I look younger than I did before and I get noticed. That's the magic of colour.

PSYCHOLOGICALLY SPEAKING

There are times in our lives when we can become anxious or nervous. It might be a presentation to the board, an interview, a blind date, meeting your daughter's boyfriend for the first time and so on. We could all do with a little help on these occasions - without hitting the gin bottle.

You may not be aware of it, but colour is a powerful medium when it comes to tackling everyday situations. You may even be wearing a colour which sends out a signal, albeit subconsciously. Pink, for instance, is thought to be the colour of love, so wearing it may be an attempt to surround ourselves with love or even attract love into our lives. I've seen many of my recently divorced clients wearing pink, even though they may have never worn it beforehand.

Think about situations that might cause anxiety in your life, or occasions when you need to be motivated or inspired. Using the following guide, discover how wearing a particular colour can help and assist you when you most need it. The colour does not have to apply to the entire outfit, sometimes just a splash will do the trick.

RED: Red has the longest wavelength, so we see it first (think traffic lights, brake lights and so on). It is stimulating and courageous. Wear it if you want to be noticed, powerful, assertive or strong. Politicians often wear a red tie when they have something important to say. The red imitates the colouring in the lips so you will automatically look at the mouth.

ORANGE: A mixture of yellow and red symbolising passion, abundance and fun. Beware though, unless you are deeply tanned, not many of us carry off this colour well. So wear as an accent colour unless you want to be Tango'd!

YELLOW: An emotional colour that governs extroversion, friendliness, creativity and optimism. It represents our personal power and how we feel about ourselves. A spot of yellow can go along way to making you feel more confident. This colour looks better on those of you with darker skins, so beware of overdoing it.

GREEN: The least worn colour in the UK, perhaps because of its 'unlucky' connotations. Green signifies balance, compassion and understanding. A useful colour to wear if you have a difficult client, a confrontation or an apology to make. Also useful to enable balance within if you feel 'out of sorts'. Bright lime green suits very few people and can reflect back onto the face giving a green shadow around the jaw. Unless you want to look like an alien, choose a darker or softer alternative.

BLUE: Governs speech, communication, creative expression and intellect. Wear it when presenting a speech or if you need a clear thought pattern. A serene and soothing colour, it mentally calms. Interestingly, Tony Blair and George W Bush both wore dark navy suits during the Iraq crisis. The message – 'trust us, we know what we are doing'. Blue worn around the throat area can help you to say what you need to say with ease.

PURPLE: A spiritual colour which is also thought to represent authenticity, truth and luxury (Cadbury's Dairy Milk was perceived to be very expensive chocolate due to its purple wrapper). It has many links with royalty and the church due to its expensive price-tag years ago.

PINK: Love and femininity. A soothing colour which radiates warmth and love. If you have a warm skin, choose coral instead of pink.

BROWN: Earthy and reliable, though can be construed as dull. Is warmer and softer than black and can look more flattering on warmer skins. For maximum impact, stick to darker shades. Wear if you want to elicit trust and openness.

BLACK: Everyone's favourite 'safe' bet. Exudes sophistication, glamour, efficiency, authority and security. Often worn as a slimming aid (though this does not work for everyone) it can drain and become serious. Wear with caution unless you know it suits you.

WHITE: White is a total reflection and represents purity. Can be perceived as hygienic and sterile which is why it's used in hospitals and clinics worldwide.

GREY: A neutral colour. Grey can have a dampening effect on other colours and can indicate a lack of confidence. However, charcoal grey may be a great alternative for suits if black is too harsh for you.

Your clothes can also have an effect when you need to modify others' perception of you to get the best result.

If you're unsure of what to wear for a particular event or occasion then take some time to complete the following exercise.

EXERCISE

First of all I'd like you to think about your own personality. Where would you sit on a scale of 1-10 with shy at 1 and very bold at 10? What do you need to be for this particular occasion? Would it be beneficial to move up or down the scale to appear more or less demanding?

The way you put your clothes together can help you to achieve a different perception of yourself by others.

One of my clients is a teacher. She works in a school where discipline is often difficult to achieve. She is expected to get great results at GCSE and, on the whole, she achieves this with hard work and dedication. She had begun to notice that recently, her pupils were taking little notice of what she was saying or doing. Her control of the class was diminishing and it was causing her distress.

We looked at her chosen style of dress. She was wearing a full length 'boho' skirt with lots of layers, teamed with a logo'd t-shirt, gold belt and flip-flop type sandals. She looked extremely trendy and the look suited both her figure and her personality. However, by dressing in this way, she looked more like one of her pupils rather than their teacher.

We needed to create a look that was still modern and up to date but also said, 'Listen to me'. I suggested she wore trousers with a matching waistcoat and a victoriana blouse in a contrasting colour. We teamed this with a pair of boots and we pinned back her hair. The result – she still felt trendy but her class instantly knew that she was in charge. No more authority problems for her.

Whether or not you work for a living, it is crucial to your well-being that you have great relationships with other people. Apparently, 85% of our problems are caused by people that we don't see eye to eye with and that's a huge potential for distress. The way you dress can once again come to your assistance. So here are some tips that will help you dress appropriately for an interaction with someone else:

✓ Authority is gained by wearing clothes with maximum contrast: black and white, dark brown and cream, navy and palest blue.

✓ A softer image is gained by dressing in different values of a single colour: brown or grey trousers and slightly lighter shade for the upper body.

✓ Plain, bold colour is authoritative.

✓ Introduce pattern or design for a softer look.

✓ A jacket that complements, but doesn't exactly match your trousers or skirt will appear less authoritative.

✓ Fabrics that are stiff and starchy will appear more authoritative than those that have more fluidity and drape. The same applies to garments with lots of fitted tailoring (authority) and less structure (approachable). A cardigan/twinset worn with trousers or a skirt will show less authority than a suit as it has no collar.

✓ Red and/or black can look powerful. Pastels will appear less so.

✓ Hairstyles that are severe will give an impression of power. The same applies to your spectacles. Black rimmed glasses are more authoritative than rimless ones.

WORDS OF WISDOM

✓ Dress for your colouring, your shape and your personality but also take into account the occasion and your audience's expectations.

✓ You don't have to be 'mutton dressed as lamb' but you do need to be modern.

✓ If you don't suit a tan, don't wear one. You've no need to keep up with the Joneses now, be your own person.

Let's Face It

"There are no ugly women. Every woman is a Venus in her own way."

BRIGITTE BARDOT

Your face is probably the most important part of your body. It's often the first thing we notice about someone, whether in a business meeting or across a crowded room.

If you're like me, you'll probably only notice the 'bad' bits of your own face. Your concentration will be on whether you have more wrinkles, bags under your eyes or spots.

Understanding the shape of your face and your features will help you to flatter what nature gave you. This in turn will enhance your natural beauty and good looks. You'll be able to choose hairstyles, specs and jewellery that really do you justice and keep you looking up to date.

Whatever your face shape, the biggest hint I can give you to looking beautiful is to SMILE. If you can't do this because you have unsightly teeth, please get them fixed. Some dentists even provide you with 3D goggles so you can watch a film while you're having work done. No excuses.

As we get older it pays to take a bit of a softer approach when it comes to hair. For drama, some women look fantastic with a short, spiky cut in a block colour but they also have the right facial features and a personality to match. Hair that is overly long can look 'girly' and dated so be aware of that if you're holding onto 20 years' growth. Softer is more flattering so if you have naturally curly hair, work with it instead of trying to straighten it. Hair should frame your face and suit your lifestyle, so bear that in mind when you're choosing a style.

To check what will really work well on you we need to go back to the art of illusion again by looking at your face's proportions. If your face is very narrow and long, it helps if we can make it appear wider. Conversely, if it's as wide as its long (square) we need to lengthen it. If it's neither of these, you can pretty well wear whatever you choose in terms of hairstyles of spectacles.

LONG FACES

Best suit hairstyles that provide some width. A high ponytail or lots of hair on top of the head will only add to the illusion of length, as will very long straight hair. Create balance by having more hair at the sides of your face or curling the hair out and away from the face. Use blow-drying to add volume at the sides. If your jaw is pointed, hair will look great if wide at this point as it will balance the face.

Spectacles and sunglasses should fit outside the contours of the face. This provides a horizontal line which shortens and widens.

If you also have a long nose, choose plastic rather than metal frames. The thicker, dark bridge will shorten the nose.

Avoid long dangly earrings as these will also drag the eye downwards. Look for earrings that are wide and sit at ear level but don't pull on the earlobe.

WIDE FACES

Need to look longer so hairstyles with height on the top or length at the bottom will achieve this. Square jaws can be complemented by longer styles and a side fringe. A jaw-length bob and a straight fringe can appear a little like curtains round a window frame.

Spectacles should sit inside the contours of the face. A high bridge in metal will lengthen the nose if required.

Earrings that are long and dangly, or hoops that appear long when viewed from the front will add required length to the face. Longer style earrings should only be worn with an open collar or neck area.

On the whole, general style principles apply just as they did to your body shape. If you have an angular face, think stiff fabrics around the neck, geometric shaped glasses and sharp haircuts. Contoured faces need more softness and look good with wavier hair, slightly curved frames and softer fabrics round the neck.

As I have a very long face, I use my oversize spectacles to shorten.

It's also interesting to note that a neckline which exactly follows the shape of the lower half of your face will be the most flattering

To find where the lowest point of your neckline should be, measure from your hairline to your chin. Take this measurement from your chin down your body. Where it lands is your 'balance point'. It's the optimum place for a pendant to sit, the top button of a jacket/cardigan to be located and where the lowest point of a neckline should sit.

EYE, EYE

If you are a spectacle wearer, you need to be aware that your whole look can rest on how well these suit you. Glasses can add impact or be almost invisible if they are frameless.

I need to wear glasses all the time so I have a variety of pairs. These are a very important accessory for me so it makes sense that I would want to vary what I wear according to how I feel and what I want to achieve.

The shape of your specs depends on your face shape, the type of frame, how much 'room' you have and the colour you choose for your individual complexion. An angular face will suit geometric frames. A rounder face will need frames that have a slight curve. This also applies to sunglasses. It's hard for someone with a short, wide face to carry off bold frames as they take over completely. You need space in your face to wear such a bold look so it screams chic not geek. If you are small in the face, opt for rimless or a very thin metallic frame. Generally speaking, if you have cool skin you will suit silver, black, blue, purple or burgundy frames. If you're a warm skinned person, you'll look better in gold, tortoiseshell, brown or red. Metal frames with a high bridge will elongate the nose. Plastic frames with a solid bridge will make the nose look shorter.

Think about what you want your glasses to say about you and choose accordingly. The bolder frames can be more fashionable and/or more authoritative. More discreet frames are just that.

Lenses that change colour according to the light used to scream 'old fashioned' and I have to say that I'm not a big fan, but there are some more subtle ones on the market now. If your eyes are sensitive to light, take a look, they may be just what you need.

I'm short-sighted but have reached that age where I can read better without my glasses. This means that soon, I will either need two separate pairs or varifocals. I did try them out a couple of years ago but felt like I was drunk. You have to move your entire head to see anything rather than just your eyes – extremely hard work. I'm obviously too quick. If you too need to go down this avenue, make sure you buy them without that telltale line in the centre of the lens. In the meantime, if you can think of anything to help me overcome this dilemma, please let me know.

There is a new independent optician just opened in my town that boasts a full-length mirror – hurrah! You really do need one to check that your glasses look right as part of the overall picture. The usual High Street chains just haven't got this yet!

WORDS OF WISDOM

✓ If you haven't changed your specs for a couple of years, you may be in danger of looking dated or frumpy. There are so many styles to choose from now and many opticians offer a second pair free. There is really no excuse not to try on some new styles and update your look.

✓ If you just need reading glasses, there are some fantastic ones on the shelves of pharmacists and supermarkets, so there's no need to spend a fortune on looking great.

✓ Bright eyewear can date very quickly and look garish. Choose darker colours or metallics to remain more current for longer.

✓ Coloured contacts can be fun but work with your own colouring for best effect.

Hair Today, Gone Tomorrow

"I think the most important thing woman can have - next to talent of course - is her hairdresser."

JOAN CRAWFORD

A few years ago, after having my own colours analysed, I decided that my highlighted golden blonde hair had got to go. As someone with cool skin the warm tones, though supposedly youthful, were not doing me any favours, especially as I cannot wear yellow on my body without looking decidedly ill. I tried various shades of ash blonde but it was a bit wishy-washy, and my true colour of mousy brown was a definite 'no no'. Desperate measures were called for.

Enter the platinum silver me. As soon as it was done, the compliments came thick and fast. Don't get me wrong, the upkeep is tremendous work and lots of money but it is definitely worth the trouble. I also feel that, when the time comes, my transition to grey hair will be less obvious than if I had stayed golden or gone brunette.

Long before TV, movies and magazines, portraits show that women were dying their hair blonde. Women's desire to look like the proverbial Barbie, young, small waist, large breasts, long blonde hair and blue eyes is a direct response to attract the male. Throughout the generations, men have been genetically disposed to prefer younger women because they tend to be healthier and so more fertile. Blonde hair changes with age. Young girls with light blonde hair become women with brown hair, which eventually will turn grey. Thus, men who prefer to date blonde women are unconsciously attempting to mate with 'younger' (therefore, healthier and more fecund) women.

Another indicator of health is physical attractiveness, which includes lustrous, shiny hair. Grey hair becomes duller, thicker and more wiry and is unlikely to look glossy. The feeling can be that, as women, we are less attractive at this stage of our lives so we use colour as camouflage. Grey-haired men, of course, are seen as distinguished but even some of them are reaching for the bottle.

Bearing this in mind, I was quite surprised by the findings of a new book 'Going Gray' by first-time author Anne Kreamer. Having had a reality check by means of a photograph taken at the age of 49, she realised that her dyed brunette long hair no longer suited her. The book catalogues her journey to ditch the colour and become friends with her natural grey. It's quite an emotional roller coaster.

We forget that only a few years ago, it was considered 'cheap' to dye your hair - remember the Clairol advert "Does she or doesn't she?" Only famous sirens of the movie screen would dare to wear obvious colour in their hair. Nowadays, nearly everyone I know, including some men, wouldn't dream of going 'au naturel'. Think also, how much revenue hairdressers would lose if we all decided to stick with our real colour.

Anne Kreamer's book intimates there are two camps - for and against dying your hair. So what's your line -

will you or won't you go grey when the time comes? According to the book, the author finds she is more attractive to the opposite sex when grey, so perhaps we need to adjust our thinking. Grey, not blonde, is the new young. Sounds good to me.

Whatever you decide, your hair is always on show. I think it's fair to say that if we have a bad hair day, our whole life is put on hold. We know logically that it will grow again but it seems that it might take a lifetime to do so.

How long is it since you had a good look at your hair? Is the style current? Does it suit you or have you not changed it for a number of years? Do you have it coloured or highlighted? Is it manageable? Does it suit your lifestyle?

A good hairdresser will ask all of these questions and more. To ensure that the hair is in proportion to your height, a professional hairstylist should ask you to stand up before making any decisions about the style and cut. They should also take into account your skin tones. Many try to 'warm you up' with gold, bronze and auburn when in fact you need ash tones to complement your cooler skin.

If you have contoured features or naturally wavy hair, you can really suit a softer style. If you have cheekbones and are more angled, you can sport a sharper look but be careful it's not so sharp that it ages you. A long, thin face can benefit from hair with width. A short, wide face needs height on top or a longer length to create slimness and length.

Notice the texture of your hair. If it's going grey and is very dry, it might benefit from a shorter cut. We all aspire to lustrous, long locks but if we haven't got them there are other ways to make your hairstyle work for you. Long hair can be ageing on some people and a short, sassy cut can take years off your general appearance. If you wear your hair up all the time – or it's very fine- ask for a short, layered cut to add volume. Longer layers on top will be more versatile. A bob is easy to manage and celebrity-led updates to this classic style means it never goes out of date. Colour, in the form of highlights or lowlights, can really add some dramatic impact and brighten up your style.

Whatever you decide, work with what you've got or you'll be forever at the mercy of your hair, and lining the pockets of your hairdresser. If you only have five minutes in the morning, don't be tempted to opt for high maintenance, however promising it sounds.

Remember, you are unique. You are no longer beholden to trends and fads. Make your hair the style everyone else fantasises about because it looks so good on you.

If you are losing your hair due to the menopause or illness, the most important thing to do is make sure that you have a really good cut. Long hair tends to drag and will pull on the scalp making the hair loss appear worse. A shortish style, perhaps with some length on the top of the head if required, will minimise the exposure. Keep the application of hair products to a minimum. Too much wax will add weight to the hair shaft and make the problem worse. Buy the very best product you can afford to thicken the hair and then use sparingly. Colour can also help. A tint or semi-permanent colour can add gloss and shine so the hair appears fuller.

Anyone can look more stylish and trendy by the introduction of a few colour highlights, some wax to give lift or a choppy cut to give a funky look. It doesn't have to take oodles of time. - a few minutes daily effort can take years off you. I'm terrible with hair so I have worn it short for years. No curling tongs or straightening irons have ever graced my dressing table. I blast it with a hairdryer and apply some wax. Stylish and funky in five minutes flat.

You can make the most of your hair by pampering yourself. There are products on the market that act like a mask, providing intensive moisture to make the hair shaft look sleek and shiny. Buy shampoos and conditioners that suit your hair type and try to wash your hair on a daily basis using a mild shampoo so it doesn't strip oils from the hair. Massaging your scalp can bring much needed blood to the surface of the scalp. Not only is this therapeutic but it will enhance the condition of your hair. As we age, the condition of our scalp can deteriorate. Follicles can become clogged, resulting in thinner hair. The scalp should be treated to an occasional mask, just like our face, if we want to keep it in tiptop condition.

The biggest problem hairdressers recognise about an 'older' woman is that they have the same hairstyle for decades. If you are suffering from a time warp where your hair is concerned, do yourself a favour and book a free consultation now. Ask for recommendations from friends or colleagues who have hair that always looks good. You don't have to go to an expensive salon. Some are trained to provide the latest celeb styles rather than what actually suits you. Many of the best hairdressers I've come across are mobile, and consequently, very affordable.

Check out other women who have hair to die for and find out where they go. If possible, accompany them to their next appointment and observe – be curious. Does the stylist listen to what the client is saying? Does each client look great in their own right or is each hairstyle similar to the next one?

If this isn't available to you, book a free consultation with three different salons. To make the best decision about which one to use, you must be armed with the correct knowledge. Your hair is your shining glory and NOTHING, NOTHING is worse than a bad hair month – even adult acne can be disguised, bad hair cannot so do your homework.

Tell them what you like/don't like and any quirks of your hair – "I always have a fringe", "my hair goes frizzy if it gets damp". If they disagree, move on. You are looking to build a relationship and that means they must respect your opinions. By all means take in pictures from magazines. Be truthful about how much time you have to do your hair. It's no good coming out of the salon looking like a million dollars if it takes an hour every morning to recreate the style and you're a 'wash'n'go' type of gal. Once you've found your stylist, hang onto him/her at all costs but be aware that even the best relationships don't always last and be prepared to move on when the time comes. The relationship with your hairdresser is precious. Trust is vital. If you find you're not resonating anymore, don't feel afraid to visit someone else. You won't regret it.

One of my clients has very long, naturally curly hair and two small children to look after as a single mother. She was promoted at work but felt her hair wasn't matching the job description. We went to a hairdresser who really listened to what she asked for and provided her with five different styles that added polish, worked well on unwashed hair and all could be achieved in under five minutes. That's a great hairdresser.

WIGS

Unfortunately, with age may come the onset of any number of illnesses, cancer being one that appears to be growing at an alarming rate. Chemotherapy can cause the hair to shed so if you don't want to remain bald, you can either cover up with a scarf or wear a wig.

There are two types of wig:

1. Handmade: light, comfortable and expensive

2. Machine Made: strips of hair are sewn onto pieces of fabric so they become bulkier and heavier to wear.

They can be made of human hair or synthetics. The latter is heavier to wear and pre styled. The former is just like your own hair and will need washing and styling.

We've all seen ladies (and men for that matter) wearing obvious wigs so here is how to ensure yours looks like your own hair:

✓ Go to the best wig centre you can find. Check with cancer specialists, hospitals, hairdressers or other cancer sufferers for referrals.

✓ Make sure it fits properly. If the staff don't know how to fit it, move on. Wear it behind your normal hairline. It must be comfortable to wear so leave it on for at least ten minutes.

✓ Stick with your own natural colour and a style that is similar to the one you normally have. Many wigs have much more hair than we would naturally have so thinning can be done by a hairdresser while it's on the stand. Any final cutting should be carried out while you are wearing it.

✓ Don't use hairspray or gel or it becomes too stiff.

WORDS OF WISDOM

✓ Softer is probably better as we age so unless you know for sure you can carry a dramatic style, think feminine.

✓ Spend time looking after your hair and it will work well for you.

✓ Bad hair is the worst thing you can ever encounter so choose your hairdresser with care.

✓ Work with what you've got not what you would like to have.

✓ Unless you can afford to visit your hairdresser more than once a week, be realistic about the time and effort you can spare to do your hair and choose your style accordingly.

Let's Kiss & Make Up

"The best thing is to look natural, but it takes make-up to look natural."

CALVIN KLEIN

I'm pretty sure that our postman thinks that my husband has two different women living at our house. Normally, he arrives very early with our mail, about 6.30am, and I am the one who goes to collect it from him. The sight must be quite frightening actually – hair standing on end like I've just electrocuted myself, eye bags like a Bassett Hound and the wrinkles of a Staffordshire Bull Terrier – no disrespect to any dogs out there. I remember vividly the day he came later than usual with a parcel to be signed for. By this time I was dressed and fully made up. When I opened the door, he stepped back in amazement and nearly dropped his packages. His eyes said it all – this *cannot* be the same woman.

I could have got very upset about this. I am well aware of how old my skin is looking. Too many years of sunbathing with olive oil and lemon juice, poor eating habits, alcohol, cigarettes, an early widowhood and stress have all shown up in my face.

I once visited a face reader. She told me that the horizontal lines on my forehead were signs of mental agility and curiosity (that word again!) for life. My eyes showed natural enthusiasm, openness, tolerance and that I was easy to get along with. As you can imagine, I liked her a lot!

Well dear reader, if I can turn myself around, so can you. We can all scrub up well if we know what we are doing. I'm not advocating that you should wear make up all the time. A beautician friend of mine never wears makeup while she's working. She has niched herself as a 'holistic' beautician and she is very successful. If you too have great skin and know you look attractive au naturel, just use this chapter for those special occasions. You may need to know, however, that research has shown that women who wear carefully applied make up for work do tend to earn up to 23% more than their bare faced colleagues, so think on.

PAINT A PICTURE

It's unfortunate, but as we get older, our skin loses colour, develops age spots and sun damage pigmentation, it sags and it wrinkles. That's a fact. It doesn't mean that the world has ended. These days, cosmetic houses are working hard to produce creams and cosmetics to suit a more mature complexion. Light-diffusing foundations, moisturising lipsticks and lip-glosses can all help create the illusion of young, healthy skin. Add to that primers, which enable make up to glide on smoothly, and fillers, which literally fill in your lines, and we don't have to look as old as we might feel.

As a rule of thumb, the following basic principles will enable you to apply your makeup in a way that enhances your complexion.

FOUNDATION

Foundation is probably the hardest item to buy correctly. It is the basis of all your makeup and is used to even out your skin tone, NOT to add colour to it. Buy only after you have seen it on your skin in broad daylight. A beautician friend of mine always says that you would never buy a shoe by trying it on your hand. It's the same with foundation. It should be placed around jaw level, not on your hand, as the skin there is totally different in colour and texture. Wait for a few minutes to let it absorb. There should be no discernible difference.

Apply your foundation all over the skin including the eye area. This will enable any eye shadow to stay in place for longer. Make sure it is well blended into the skin, especially around the jaw and hairline. If you want a more natural look, you can blend it with moisturiser, or use a damp sponge or foundation brush to give less coverage. I find it covers more naturally if you start from the centre of the face and blend outwards. This way you have less left on the sponge or your fingertips when you reach your hairline. There is nothing worse than seeing too much depth of colour in the hair or at jaw level.

You may find that, like me, you have different coloured skin on your neck, chin, cheeks and forehead so a sole foundation doesn't always work. You may need to use concealer first or just use foundation on some of your skin. Prescriptives now sell Custom Blend foundations, which match your skin perfectly and they'll whip one up according to what your own skin needs in terms of moisture level, coverage and so on. It costs about £40, so well worth tracking down. Most cosmetic houses sell light-diffusing foundations that are supposed to make us look younger. They are light in texture but still give a good coverage. I like Bobbi Brown's products as she herself is in her 50s and I believe she really understands what we need at this age. Heavier foundations can sit in the wrinkles of the skin so beware.

CONCEALER

Used to hide blemishes and dark under-eye circles, it can be a godsend if applied correctly. I always apply before my foundation, because my skin is very mottled and I find it evens it out. If you have a blemish you want to hide you may the foundation has done the job well enough, so apply any concealer afterwards.

For under-eye circles, use a light creamy formulation so it won't drag the delicate skin under the eye. Dab it on using a concealer brush or your ring finger, as it has less power than your index finger and you don't want to poke your eye out. For optimum effect, layer on two tones. Start with a lighter, pinkish one to neutralise the darkness and cover with a yellow, flesh toned one. Make sure you blend well. This also works well for spider veins if you use a fine brush to apply and your fingers to blend.

If you have high colour, a green cream will disguise the redness. This will also work on pimples that are red and angry looking. Don't choose one that is too greasy or it will make the problem worse.

Darker spots or moles need a heavier consistency. A stick or pencil is your best choice.

POWDER

Buy a fine, translucent powder as a setting agent. Dab over your face with the powder puff. Remove excess by using a large brush with downward strokes. If you have wrinkles, buy the finest texture you can find otherwise it will show up in the lines on your face. If you want a tanned effect, use a bronzer with a large brush and sweep over the face and neck – lightly being the operative word here.

Unfortunately, my face is unevenly pigmented due to the sunbathing I overdid in my 30s. I cannot wear foundation all over my face but have to stop before I hit my chin and jawline otherwise I have a tidemark. To even it out, I use a really fine colourless powder, so it doesn't sit in any wrinkles, and blend concealer onto any noticeable blemishes. This has taken years to get right and I am very grateful to my friend and colleague Patrick Swan for his help. As a make-up artist to the stars, including Madonna, and a TV presenter to boot I'm in very good hands. Visit *www.patrickswan.com* for more information.

If you are suffering from hot flushes you may want to try Bourjois Anti-Shine Blotting Sheets or use tissues to blot up any excess moisture. Re-apply foundation and use powder to set as appropriate.

BLUSHER

You can find both cream and powder blushers on the market. I tend to stick with a fine powder as the cream doesn't seem to stay put on me. Cream blushers can be more youthful though, so if you don't mind reapplying throughout the day, this is your best bet.

To apply powder blusher, smile. Using a brush, start from the apple of your cheek and blend upwards and backwards towards the hairline. To ensure you're not heavy handed, hold the brush loosely between thumb and 1st and 2nd fingers and not as if you were holding a pencil (like Groucho Marx and his cigar) and shake any excess onto a tissue before application. For a special evening look, lightly brush the forehead, nose and chin with blusher to highlight the T zone. If you are using cream, you can use your fingers.

EYEBROWS

Eyebrows act as a frame for your face. Take a pencil and hold by the side of your nose, lining it up to the inner corner of your eye. Where the tip ends is where your eyebrow should start. Keeping the pencil by your nose, move the pencil tip towards the outer corner of your eye and this indicates where your brow should end. Take a grey or brown pencil (or use eyeshadow and a brush) and use feather like strokes to fill in any gaps. If you are using powder, go against the direction of hair growth for best results.

Make sure you keep your eyebrows in good shape, either by plucking, waxing or threading. Really unruly eyebrow hairs can be professionally removed by electrolysis. Always remove stray hairs from the bottom and never the top of the brow. Pull skin tautly between your fingers and tweeze out in the direction of the hair growth. It's often a good idea to colour in the perfect eyebrow first. This will provide a template so stray hairs can be easily spotted. Clear mascara can help keep unruly hairs in place.

Once again I messed up. I had eyebrows that would have competed with those of Dennis Healey when I was young. In those days, eyebrows were plucked out and replaced by a pencilled arch. I wasn't brave enough to be unique at the age of eleven – you just want to be the same as your peers – so I plucked them out every day. Eventually they wouldn't grow at all and looked awful.

So I took radical action and had them tattooed back on. I had heard many reports of semi-permanent make up not going as well as planned, so I had walked away from it as a possible solution. I then bumped into a friend who told me about Denise Collinson. My friend had a semi-permanent eyeliner applied and it looked great. Denise is very professional and you trust her immediately. She actually lowered my brows so that my eyes now look enormous. You do need some high-end maintenance the first week as you can't let your brows get wet. This can be problematical if you have a power shower but my husband jumped to the rescue and bought me some welder's safety goggles. Don't even think about it! It did work but looking for the shampoo was bordering on dangerous at times. You also need to sleep on your back so that any flaking remains at a minimum. The colour can look quite dark to start with but it does fade and you can have top-ups free of charge within the first three months if you need to. So here I am, with lovely eyebrows, and it really didn't hurt – thanks Denise. You can contact her and look at some of her work at *www.denisecollinsonpermanentmakeup.co.uk*

Eye shadow looks better if it's not too pearly or iridescent, as these can highlight any wrinkling. Bright greens and blues should be left to the young. Try neutral colours with a brighter eye pencil to add interest. Eye pencils should be applied with light, feathery strokes to define the area underneath the eye and in the outer corners. You can use a strong eye shadow and brush if you prefer. There are many mineral based powder shadows and blushers around at the moment. They are supposed to be pure enough to sleep in but I wouldn't like to risk it – plus it creates more washing. They do apply really well on more mature skins, look very natural and do a good job of concealing any blemishes.

Finish the look with a coat of mascara. Unless you're very dark, avoid black and opt for grey or black/brown. Many cosmetic houses now do stunning shades of turquoise and purple if you want a different and dramatic look.

To use mascara to its best advantage, look down and lightly brush the top side of your upper lashes first. This will provide length. Then looking straight at the mirror, brush the underside upwards.

If you wear mascara on your lower lashes, use a zigzag motion with the wand first. Then you can brush downwards to get length and volume if required. Don't be too heavy handed with your application on the lower lashes or they might end up looking like spider's legs – very dating. The current trend is to make your eyes almond shaped rather than round.

If your eyelashes are sparse, use an eyelash conditioner first. This will provide moisture and add thickness. If they are very straight, use an eyelash curler to open up the eye area, before applying your mascara.

f you have eyes set wide apart, your eye pencil should run two thirds of the lower lid, working from the outer corner. If they are narrow set, use only one third and blend well. This will make the eyes appear to be spaced wider apart. Always remember to blend using a cotton bud so the line appears softer. Harsh lines are very ageing.

If you have little or no eyelids, dispense with eyeliner on your top lids. It will make the eyelids look heavy and you will look tired. Use a lighter colour instead to open them up. An alternative is to apply eyeliner under the rim of your top eyelid. This is a trick I learned From Frey-Ja Barker, Fenwicks 020 7409 9824. To do this safely, you need to affect a 'shocked' look so your eyes become wide open (like headlights). Take a flat brush and apply gel eyeliner (Bobbi Brown has a wide selection) to the rim, pushing it into your lashes. It is very dramatic and shows off the whites off your eyes beautifully.

A prominent browbone should not be highlighted with a light colour as it will make it stand out even more. Instead use a colour that almost matches your skin tone so it recedes.

If you wear specs don't make the mistake of piling on the eye makeup to compensate. Check whether your eyes look smaller or larger when you have your glasses on. If smaller, line your eyes both top and bottom to make them stand out more. If larger, blend, blend, blend and don't be heavy handed. Glasses will always draw attention to your eyebrows, so make sure they are perfectly groomed.

LIPS

Our lip lines often get blurred as we age and if you smoke you may find that lipstick 'bleeds' into tiny cracks around your mouth creating feathery lines. This is especially true of lip gloss. There are special products on the market to counteract this and they are well worth investing in. Body Shop does a great one for about £7 (Body Shop Lip Fixer) and it contains beeswax to soften and keep lips moist. I also like Guerlain's Lip Lift as it helps to plump up lips and keeps your lipstick 'fixed' all day.

Your lip line may get thinner. If so, don't choose a lip colour that is too dark as it will make them look even smaller. To outline the lip area, choose a lip pencil that is close to your own lip colour, rather than one that matches your lipstick. This will provide a better outline and can make the lips look larger if required. Don't try to draw the lip outline in one go, as it will often look clownish. Break it down into stages. Firstly, draw in your cupid's bow. Then take the pencil and draw in the equivalent distance on your bottom lip. You can then connect the dots moving from the centre to the corner of the mouth. You may find that you only need to do part of this. If you already have a full bottom lip, don't bother drawing it in, stick to the top one only.

Use a lip brush to apply your lipstick or gloss. To keep lipstick on your lips, blot with a tissue and then re-apply. You could opt for a semi permanent lipline, courtesy of Denise Collinson or other professionals in this field, if you feel that this is something that would enhance your looks.

If your lips are particularly chapped, use a mild exfoliator to remove any dead skin. Otherwise the lipstick will not sit properly. You need to prepare your lips just like you would prepare a wall before applying wallpaper.

Remember to choose cosmetics that suit your complexion and your colouring (see the chapter called 'Face Facts'). Opt for rose tones if cool and coral if warm. If you are dark, you can wear deeper shades than if you are fair (but beware, they can show up dark eye circles). If you are bright, you can wear brighter lipstick. If muted, stick to softer shades. But remember, light shades will always enlarge and dark, reduce. Where we might want to wear dark trousers to slim down large hips, it's probably the opposite for your lips. For once bigger is better. Plump lips equal youthfulness. So why not be curious, investigate some new lipstick choices and see what reaction you get.

You can sometimes go a little warmer in your makeup choices if you are 'medium' colouring or on the borderline of warm/cool as it can help you look younger but experiment and gauge reactions before changing everything overnight.

Don't be intimidated by sales assistants on the cosmetics counters. Many are on commission, so ask their advice but don't feel you have to buy. As many department stores have terrible lighting and are situated in covered shopping centres, you won't get an accurate picture of yourself. Find an assistant who you like the look of – perhaps she is older or she wears less makeup – and book an appointment with her in the daytime, explaining exactly what you hope to achieve and any problems you have. Before you make any purchase, go home and look at your new look in your own mirror. This way, you'll be able to compare the old with the new before making expensive mistakes. Alternatively, ask for samples of what they've used do you can try it yourself at home.

If you're worried that you'll be 'sold to' or you want a little more privacy, both Frey-Ja Barker and Patrick Swan undertake private consultations with no allegiance to any specific brands. They have access to a very wide range of skin care products and cosmetics so can help you choose what is best for you, your personality, your lifestyle and your budget.

EVENING MAKEUP

At night we need more colour not more makeup. So add slightly deeper or brighter shades to your lips, eyes and cheeks. Apply using dim light rather than bright fluorescence which is too harsh. Apply daytime make up in natural light if you can.

CLEANSING

I have no wish to teach grandmothers to suck eggs so to speak, so forgive me if your cleansing routine has been maintained for years. It becomes even more important as we get older and your oestrogen levels change, that you don't skimp on looking after your skin. Cleanse, tone and moisturise with products suitable for your skin type at least once a day. This will help you to retain the dewiness and freshness of younger skin. One with SPF15 minimum will prevent further damage from the sun. Lastly, ALWAYS take off your makeup before going to bed, without rubbing at the delicate skin around your eyes. Who wants to wake up to dirty pillowcases?

Talking of pillowcases, I have been reliably informed that silk ones prevent the face wrinkling from sleep and also keep your hairstyle intact. You'll have to test that one out for yourself. It's also said that sleeping on your back is better for your complexion. Sleeping on your side creases the face and encourages wrinkles. I have tried this on a couple of occasions (being curious) and have to say, I did look better in the morning. There was a price to pay though in terms of comfort – foetal position is so much nicer. The other major problem with lying on your back is it does encourage snoring – usually very loud - or it does in the case of my husband anyway!

If you so desire, you can use a facemask after exfoliating on a weekly basis. Be careful if your skin is delicate or very dry that the exfoliating scrub is not too harsh for your skin. I often apply vitamin E oil as I feel that it sinks into my skin and nourishes it really well. If you do it prior to going to sleep, you wake up with gorgeously soft skin.

Then close the pores by using a non-astringent toner or splash your face with cold water if you prefer.

Before moisturising, you may want to use a repair serum, to deliver a rich dose of anti-oxidants and sun protection. Many claim to prevent age spots but mine haven't disappeared yet. It is however, crucial to wear at least SPF 15 in either your moisturiser, serum or foundation every single day, even in winter. You may also want to use a 'filler' to fill in the lines between your wrinkles and/or a primer to ensure your make up glides on smoothly. If you're a 'wash'n'go' gal, it's OK to omit these steps as long as you ensure you are adding moisture to your skin.

Day creams tend to be lighter than night creams, as all the repair work is done while we are in bed. Be careful of putting too much around the eyes as it can make them puffy. Specialist eye creams should be used for this purpose, dabbed on the top of the cheek bone gently using the ring finger so the skin doesn't get dragged and damaged.

With fluctuating oestrogen levels, you may find that your skin will become much drier or much oilier. If this is the case, you will need to change your skin creams accordingly. It's not always the case that you have to splash out on expensive skin creams but do watch out for an overload of chemicals. I like Ren, because they are great to use and seem to use more pure ingredients than most on the market.

DARE TO BARE

Don't forget the rest of your body. A weekly exfoliate plus daily moisturising can be of great help to the skin covering the rest of you. I like Clarins, as their exfoliators turn to a lovely oil on contact with your skin. They smell divine too. If that's too much trouble, run yourself a bath and soak in some luxurious oils with a glass of champagne at your side.

Yogis are always keen to tell you that the King and Queen of asanas (postures) are the headstand and the shoulderstand, which should be performed daily for at least 25 breaths. Why? Because they allow the blood to go to the head, keeping the brain active and the skin radiant. If you're not willing to go that far, please treat yourself to a regular massage. It's really important that the lymph moves around the body and that blood gets to parts that it doesn't usually reach. De-stressing is no longer a luxury but a necessity as we get older, so make a pampering session a priority.

CELLULITE

Much has been made of cellulite – those bumpy lumps under the skin, usually around the bottom and the back of the thighs. Some doctors swear it doesn't exist but I know many people who believe differently.

If you do have these orange peel type lumps, you can try body brushing. Use a bristle body brush in circular motions, moving towards the heart. Do this before showering and hopefully, you may notice a difference. There are specialist creams on the market that you could try too. Drinking water and regular exercise may also help alleviate the problem. I'm trying hard to increase my water quota so I'll let you know how I get on. I have loved coffee all my life and it's always been my drink of choice, so once again there's a price being paid here. I'm glad to say that I stick to one a day most days and I really savour every last drop. The strange thing is that if I now over-indulge, I can't sleep, so that alone is enough of a reason to reach for the herbal tea. Green tea is a good alternative as it contains loads of anti oxidants and is supposed to increase metabolic rate too.

In terms of water, here is the definitive rule of thumb on how much you need to drink on a daily basis. Take your weight in pounds and halve it. This equals the number of fluid ounces you should be drinking each day. There are 20 fluid ounces in a pint, so you'll need to do the maths. If you weigh 10 stone, which is 140 pounds, you'll need 3.5 pints i.e. 140 divided by 2 equals 70 divided by 20 equals 3.5. Try to take water in its natural form by eating lots of fruit and vegetables as it is more easily absorbed this way – read the chapter 'Green is for Go' for more information.

STRETCH MARKS

Applying a vitamin E oil or cream can help reduce stretch marks. Don't expect miracles overnight. Your skin will feel really soft though. Bio Oil is also good for this purpose.

Make sure you also take a good mineral and vitamin supplement, especially as most food is not as fresh as one would wish for. I've found vitamin B to be most helpful especially where my moods have been concerned. As most vitamins are excreted daily, you'll need to keep up the intake. If you are menopausal, you may want to seek out a nutritionist who can help you with your diet and any other nutritional supplements you might need. Many swear by Black Cohosh, Red Clover and Wild Yam to help alleviate unpleasant symptoms such as night sweats and mood swings.

NAIL BITING

Ragged or unkempt nails can really let you down. Following the trend set in the USA, many nail bars have been set up around the country,so there is no excuse for having dodgy digits.

HOME MANICURE

✓ Soak nails for five minutes then remove existing polish with cotton wool and nail polish remover.

✓ Clip nails straight across. Pointed nails are weaker.

✓ File nails, working from outside in. They should be square with slightly rounded edges.

✓ Apply cuticle remover and soften hands in water for three minutes.

✓ Wrap cotton wool around an orange stick and GENTLY push back cuticles. Wash your hands.

✓ Apply base coat before applying nail colour and a final topcoat.

✓ If you wear acrylic nails or you polish regularly, be sure to give your own nails a breather now again. They can suffer from staining and a lack of oxygen.

✓ Feet are something we really take for granted. Think how you would manage if something happened to them and you couldn't walk. It's time to give them some recognition and a well-earned pampering session. I couldn't live without my foot spa and my feet say "thank you" too.

HOME PEDICURE

✓ Soak nails for five minutes. Take off existing polish with cotton wool and nail polish remover.

✓ Clip nails straight across and file if necessary towards the centre with single strokes.

✓ Buff the surface of the nail to remove ridges.

✓ Apply cuticle remover and soak feet for about three minutes – add lemon juice if nails are stained.

✓ Gently push back cuticles using an orange stick wrapped with cotton wool.

✓ Use an exfoliator to remove dry skin on backs of heels or soften any callouses.

✓ Dry feet thoroughly and apply a rich foot cream.

✓ Separate toes with tissue and apply base coat. When dry, apply colour and a topcoat.

✓ These days it's more youthful to wear colour on your feet and a more natural shade on your fingers. Matching your polish on hands and feet is very dated. So unless you want to create some drama for a specific occasion, ditch the bright reds and deep colours. They also show up any chips more easily too.

GIRL POWER

It is unfortunate but one of the downsides of not going grey and avoiding elasticated waistbands is that the pressure to look ever youthful is on us at every stage of our lives. We can't all look like Sharon Stone or Madonna, but not taking care of your appearance may hamper your success in all areas of your life. Attractive people have more influence in their friendships, work and partnerships. They are also more confident. Not fair but true, so you owe it yourself to make the most of what you've got. As you get older, it will get harder.

If you still need convincing that applying make up can give you a real boost, the following might help change your mind.

I work as a volunteer for a charity called Look Good Feel Better (*www.lgfb.co.uk*). They organise a number of workshops in major hospitals throughout the UK for adies who have undergone treatment for cancer. During these workshops, my colleagues and I teach the ladies how to apply make up step by step. The transformation is amazing. They not only look fantastic, but their excitement and enthusiasm levels go through the roof. The buzz in the atmosphere is tremendous. They definitely leave the room with a completely different and much more positive attitude to when they first came in. If you are a make up virgin, have a go and see what the power of make up can do for you.

WORDS OF WISDOM

✓ Less is more where make up is concerned. Stick to neutrals that flatter and blend, blend, blend.

✓ Don't skimp on skin care.

✓ Pampering is essential.

✓ Use experts for their advice but don't be bullied into buying.

✓ Spraying perfume on your neck can irritate the skin and attract sun damage. Spray on your wrists or into the air and walk through the mist.

Fashion Feng Shui®
(The Art of Dressing Your Essence & Your Intention)

"My mother says I didn't open my eyes for eight days when I was born, but when I did, the first thing I saw was an engagement ring. I was hooked."

ELIZABETH TAYLOR

It really started with a simple question. Someone asked me for my favourite colour and there was no hesitation in answering, 'indigo'. I love its rich, luxurious, bold, dynamic characteristics and always have. But on answering, I realised that if I loved it so much, why didn't I wear it?

As a qualified colour consultant, I am well aware of the importance of matching the characteristics of colour to a person's complexion so they always look radiant. As a 'summer', indigo is too dark for my skin, so I had forsaken it for lilacs, mauves and paler blues. But lilac is no match for a deep, inky purple as far as my heart is concerned, so there had to be an answer. If you really love a colour, there must be a way to wear it without looking old or tired and I was determined to find it.

Fashion Feng Shui® came to the rescue. It's an innovative, transformational dressing technique inspired by Feng Shui, the ancient Chinese Art of

Placement. Based on the premise that you live a happier, healthier, more prosperous existence when your living and working environments are harmonious and balanced, Feng Shui encourages you to visually affirm your intentions in your personal and professional surroundings in order to create them in your life.

I had always thought that Feng Shui was only applicable to your home but in reality, clothing is your body's most intimate environment. You wear clothing every day and choose it to according to the occasion, your lifestyle and your emotions. How many of us have swapped clothes because we are having a 'fat day' or we want to feel in control? How many of us have put on an outfit that has felt terrible or wonderful all day according to how we are feeling? Emotions and spirit play a large part in a way a woman dresses, otherwise we would just put on the same old things every day without caring what we look or feel like.

What you wear is as influential on your life as your home and business decors, and you need to dress with mindfulness and intention so that your clothes not only express your authenticity but can attract your deepest desires.

Take a look at the following questions and tick which one is most like you. I am:

☐ 1. Artistic, intellectual and/or non-conforming

☐ 2. Energetic, competitive and/or outdoorsy

☐ 3. Charismatic, alluring and/or fun-loving

☐ 4. Conservative, nurturing and/or a homemaker

☐ 5. Refined, organised and/or meticulous

IF YOU TICKED 1, YOU ARE A PHILOSOPHER

You like your clothes to be different. Your signature style is Creative. Choose trends that reflect **WATER** Energetic Design Elements: *Dark colours, wavy patterns; fluid or sheer fabrics; velvety textures; flowing or asymmetrical shapes; unique styling*

IF YOU TICKED 2, YOU ARE A PIONEER

You like your clothes to be comfortable. Your signature style is Sporty. Choose trends that reflect **WOOD** Energetic Design Elements: *Blues and greens; stripes or florals; natural fibre fabrics; columnar shapes; trousers; casual or athletic styling.*

IF YOU TICKED 3, YOU ARE A PLEASURE SEEKER

You like your clothes to attract attention. Your personal style is Dramatic. Choose trends that reflect **FIRE** Energetic Design Elements: *Reds and purples; pointed or angular shapes; animal prints and fabrics; attention-getting or body-conscious styling.*

IF YOU TICKED 4, YOU ARE A PEACEMAKER

You like to be conservative. Your personal style is Traditional. Choose trends that reflect **EARTH** Energetic Design Elements: *Browns; yellows and earth-tones; squared shapes; basic fabrics; nubby textures; comfortable or classic styling.*

IF YOU TICKED 5, YOU ARE A PERFECTIONIST

You like your clothes to be the best. Your personal style is Elegant. Choose trends that reflect **METAL** Energetic Design Elements: *White, pastels or metallics; rounded or arched shapes; luxurious fabrics; polished textures; elegant or designer styling.*

These represent your Essence or your core being and each one uses one of Nature's Five Elements; Water, Wood, Fire, Earth and Metal to describe physical appearance, preferences and goals, lifestyle, and clothing design elements.

By adding these elements to the way you dress, you will always be true to yourself and your essential being. For me indigo, or deep purple is a Fire element and I am fundamentally a Pleasure Seeker. On learning this, I now understood why I loved it so much and by following Feng Shui I had carte blanche to wear it. I may not always wear it close to my face but I have shoes, handbags and suede gloves as part of my regular clothing ensemble and I feel so alive when I wear them – who says handbags can't change your mood? I am also Wood and this certainly tells me why I'm never out of my jeans and am always *doing* stuff rather than just *being*. There is also a high percentage of metal in my character and this would explain why my favourite neutral is grey.

To look our best our clothing should always suit our body shape, colouring, life style and personality and this is fundamental. But what if we need to introduce a new element into our lives? If life is hectic, we need calm. If it's boring, we need excitement. What about the things we desire? To be more grounded, to have freedom, to have fun and so on. Applying the Feng Shui principles can help us, even if it's something you desire for a very short time, such as nurturing when you are feeling ill.

Here is an overview of the basic principles and how you can use them to realise your 'intention':

WATER is introspective and represents 'being'. If you want to attract more depth, quiet, stillness or tranquillity then wear clothes in black or dark tones, in an asymmetric pattern such as paisley. Fabrics should be fluid, flowing, sheer or drapey. The overall effect is undulating and soft.

WOOD is dynamic and represents 'doing'. Clothes that support this should be blue or green, columnar in shape and pattern (including vertical stripes, ribbing, corduroy) or of a floral theme. Fabrics should be crisp or springy. Jeans fit into this category extremely well. The overall effect is vertical and sporty.

FIRE is dramatic and means 'exciting'. To bring energy and radiance into your life you will need to bring out red and purple. If you can't wear red, think about introducing a handbag or shoes. Fire also embraces animal prints and diamond or triangular patterns in clingy fabrics or natural ones such as leather, fur, taffeta, wool or silk. The overall effect is angular and bold.

EARTH is traditional and represents 'nurturing'. If you need to be grounded, turn to earthy colours such as yellow and brown. Plaids, checks and boxy styles in coarse or napped textures give the feeling of being cared for. The overall effect is boxy and square with horizontal lines in the garment.

METAL stands for elegance and should be worn if you need 'refinement' in your life. As the name suggests, white, pastel and metallic colours in luxurious, shimmering fabrics are the clothes to introduce. Arched or dotty patterns suit this well. The overall effect is figure of eight and curvy.

During a consultation, you'll be given Body Colour Wands that reflect your hair, eye and skin tones. Elemental skin tones create a corporal connection and are ideal for underwear and footwear. Eye colours enhance interpersonal integrity so are best worn on the upper body, either in clothing or accessories, for maximum impact. Hair colour is worn as an outer garment or investment garment and provides overall balance. As these shades are predominantly neutral they are ideal for handbags, shoes, outerwear, skirts and trousers.

Use these guidelines in conjunction with what you know about your own style preferences and you'll soon see a difference. My own clients were sceptical at first but once they have been through the consultation, they all agreed it was life-changing. The concept of aligning the physical body with the mind and spirit is what makes this so wonderful to work with. By applying these basic principles you can elevate what was once a mundane routine to a mindful ritual, so that getting dressed becomes easy, fun AND empowering.

So when you look at the guidelines provided by the previous chapters, take note also of your Feng Shui tendencies and try to incorporate them into your every day life. If you need to take action at work, dress appropriately for your workplace and your body shape but add some wood element and you'll be sure to get the work done.

The principles of Feng Shui can be followed even further, specifically when you are purchasing clothes. Garments can retain the energy of their previous lives, so it is important to be aware of their vibrational quality and history, or provenance.

Clothes that are made from organically produced materials have more positive associations, or happy memories, attached to them. Clothes made by loving hands or socially responsible, environmentally friendly companies will have a corresponding beneficial impact on you. Those manufactured from tainted materials or in unpleasant surroundings may affect you negatively. Clothes, like food, are best when consumed as close as possible to their natural state. The less processing a garment has gone through, the fewer the opportunities it has had to pick up negative vibes along the way from its production to point-of-sale.

I was so bowled over by this concept that I became the first (and at the time of writing, the only) Fashion Feng Shui® practitioner in the UK. For more information visit *www.fashionfengshui.com* where you can buy Evana Maggiore's book, which covers this fascinating subject in far more depth. Be curious, what have you got to lose?

WORDS OF WISDOM

✓ To truly honour yourself, dress with your essence and intention in mind.

✓ To remain balanced, wear an item of clothing from each category.

✓ Think about a garment's heritage. Where did it come from? Is it ethically produced?

The Real Deal
(Putting It All Together)

"Why not be oneself? That is the whole secret of a successful appearance. If one is a greyhound, why try to look like a Pekinese?"

EDITH SITWELL

Now we get down to the real nitty-gritty. You've established your overall body and face shape, the colours that best suit you, how to disguise any figure challenges, your essence and your intentions.

This chapter is about putting it all together to ensure you understand what makes you, you. It's no good following the rules if you don't feel comfortable with the overall result. Clothes, and how you buy them, should be an extension of your personality, not a suit of armour or a mask. Don't think designer labels are the answer. It's the congruency between you and your clothing that gives you your power and not the label on show.

I have a slim, angular body and the expertise to make my legs appear much longer than they are. In theory, I would look good wearing a mini skirt and high heels. However, this style of dress does not fit in with my overall values, my personality or my age. The result – I would look and feel uncomfortable, lose my confidence and probably bolt for the nearest hiding place. This is even more alarming when you understand that 'talking' to people is one of my pleasures in life and I'm very well practised.

A client of mine works in an office environment where suits are the norm for both men and women. She is a larger than life, bubbly person and the idea of her wearing a buttoned up suit just does not sit well. Between us, we've managed to create a look that fits in with her corporate lifestyle but also expresses her own unique personality. Instead of using pin-stripes and severe tailoring in her clothing, she has selected a less structured style of suit. She wears this with brightly coloured blouses with frilly collars in soft, floaty fabrics. She looks professional, but also liberated. Her hair is left loose or pinned back, with tendrils to soften her face. She looks fantastic and radiates confidence. Guess what, she is also highly successful. Because she looks and feels confident, she attracts colleagues and clients who want to work with her. Good news for the bottom line and her promotional prospects.

STEP 1

Think about the words you would use to describe yourself. Make a list, group them and then narrow it down to two or three key adjectives. These will be your values. Take your time over this as it's the key to finding the real you.

My three Key Words are:

1...

2...

3...

STEP 2

Look at your style of dress. Does it fully express the words you've just used about yourself? If not, why not?

For instance, if one of your key descriptors is 'enthusiastic', it will come across more successfully with a wardrobe using colour rather than housing completely dark or neutral clothing. If it's 'honesty' perhaps some earthier tones may be useful.

My current style of dress is:

....

....

....

....

STEP 3

Ask someone you trust to describe you. Are the adjectives they use the same as yours? If not, ask them why they see you differently. Does your style have anything to do with it? Are your clothes giving out the wrong impression?

My friend's descriptors of me are:

1..

2..

3..

SWAP SHOP

A magazine article I once read has long stuck in my mind. Entitled 'Frock Swap', it was an article about two journalists, one from Vogue the other from The

Times, covering Paris Fashion Week but having to wear each other's clothes – how scary is that? Reading through it, it became very clear that their styles had nothing in common – how many of you would be ecstatic over a beige jumpsuit? On the other hand, being told you look like a sofa cover is not the best comment you could hope for.

The message was clear. What this article really pointed out was that it's useless to try and copy someone else's style. You may think they look great in that chiffon blouse but it doesn't mean you will too. Just imagine going to a really special occasion, a wedding maybe, in someone else's clothes. How would you feel? Uncomfortable, lacking in confidence and that's just for starters. It's making me shiver just thinking about it.

Apart from our physical attributes, we also have different personalities, lifestyles, likes and dislikes all needing accommodation in our outfits. The way we walk plays a big part, yet is often overlooked in how we choose our garments. If you have a beautiful undulating swing to your hips, think how fantastic the fluid movement of a soft, swishy hemmed skirt would be. Imagine also how restricting a pencil skirt might be on someone who moves quickly with purpose and long strides. I know, as I am that woman and have a number of ripped seams to prove it. Failing to take this into account often explains why a garment might look good on you but you never get round to actually wearing it – ring any bells? Katherine Hepburn was famous for wearing trousers in an era when they weren't fashionable for women. She has been quoted as saying *"I like to move fast, and wearing high heels was tough, and low heels with a skirt is unattractive. So pants took over."* What a savvy woman she was. She took comfort and practicality and made them her own authentic style and brand.

Clothing and the way you dress is unique for you and certainly as you get older, you owe it to yourself to find out exactly what this means. Younger people can get away with experimenting, and they should. It's part of growing up and finding out who they are. They also usually have fantastic skin, lots of attitude and a great physique so can carry more things off. When we get older, experimentation that goes wrong gets us noticed for the wrong reasons. Labels such as 'mutton dressed as lamb' or the opposite, 'frumpy', when playing it safe, can be bandied about, usually behind your back.

FINDING YOUR OWN STYLE

We are all unique and trying to copy a style just because it suits someone else is nigh on impossible. The following will help you understand the way you prefer to dress. It will also help you realise that your shopping habits and wardrobe management may be totally different from those around you.

Think about the following:

a.   Do you covet the latest trends and constantly change your look?

b.   Do you prefer quality tailoring that allows easy co-ordination of your clothes?

c.   Do you love pretty, feminine clothes and prefer skirts to trousers?

d.   Are you a 'wash'n'go' type of person who opts for a more natural, relaxed look?

e. Do you create a statement by using the unusual, such as a great piece of jewellery, a funky hairstyle or wearing clothes in strong colour combinations?

Choose the one that is most like you as it will be a key indicator of how your personality is reflected through your attire.

If you are most like answer a, then you are a **CREATIVE** dresser. The best type of shopping for you is rummaging through charity shops and vintage stores to find eclectic items which you can throw together. Chain stores hold no appeal as they are too 'mass market'. You crave individuality and artistry.

If you resonated with answer b, you are a **CLASSIC** dresser. You love garments that stand the test of time and always look smart due to their tailoring. Rarely are textures or colours mixed as you prefer a coordinated approach to dressing. You will hardly ever (if at all) be spotted wearing jeans or cords. Fashion trends do not interest you at all.

If you selected c as your answer, you love the feminine, and masculine attire does not interest you. You are a **ROMANTIC** dresser. Pretty colours, florals, patterns and floaty fabrics are the essence of your wardrobe. Your clothes may not be too structured but you will pay attention to the detail.

If you picked d as the answer most like you, then you are a **CASUAL** dresser. You may have leanings towards sporty clothes such as trainers and t-shirts, rather than high heels and blouses, or just prefer natural fabrics with little or no structure. Relaxed and comfortable are your key words. You will wear minimal jewellery and little or no makeup, with hair tied back or flowing loose around your face.

The answer e reflects a **DRAMATIC** dresser. You create attention by using unique and individual accessories or by bold use of colour. You may be high-maintenance and you may also have lots of clothes that have been worn once (you couldn't possibly wear it again – someone may have seen it before!). Clothes make a statement about you and, even if you're not aware of it, you will be noticed.

Make the most of your style by choosing garments and accessories that fit in with your natural personality.

CREATIVE dressers can choose belts, scarves that don't co-ordinate, vintage pieces, unusual brooches or corsages, crocheted shrugs, feather boas or anything that looks slightly eccentric to show off their look to the maximum. Mixing textures such as wool and chiffon can also work as long as it doesn't add unwanted bulk. Be careful not too make excessive purchases that mean items never get worn. If you want to follow the trends, make sure you adapt them to your age and body line.

CLASSIC dressers can mix and match existing garments with any new purchases. Try to vary your look by bringing in some colour. Simplicity and understatement are key to your look so beware of wearing too many pieces of jewellery at once. Although you may prefer the real thing, try good quality costume jewellery if you want to add some variety. To modernise, change your hosiery to flesh coloured fishnets or a softly patterned dark opaque. Handbags and shoes should no longer match exactly so keep the colours the same but change fabric types. Make sure that your garments are classic but not dated, if you want to look youthful.

ROMANTIC dressers can look great in garments that have some appliqué, beading or diamante. Soft layers, floaty fabrics, frills in chiffon or lace are your style. Select luxurious fabrics such as cashmere, satin and silk, for both outerwear and underwear. Soft, pretty cardigans or shrugs may look better than a jacket. Floral prints and abstracts can work well but remember your scale and don't overdo it. Woven or decorative handbags look better than stiff leather. Don't forget your heels – as if you would!

NATURAL dressers look best in natural fabrics and neutral colours. For you, linen, wool, suede, leather in loose fitting styles will make the best jackets. Choose comfortable shoes but try to make them modern – ballet pumps, for instance, can look great with jeans or a skirt. Gilets, boot cut trousers and wrap cardigans are easy to wear and can look natural and stylish at the same time. If you must have elasticated waists, make sure they don't bulk and give you bumps where you don't want them. Remember though that being relaxed does not mean not making an effort. A pair of pearl earrings, some mascara and lip-gloss can provide extra glamour when required.

DRAMATIC dressers need to look for key pieces that add impact. Wear unusual buckles on your belt, eye-catching spectacles, a huge cocktail ring, a unique bag or killer shoes. Only one or two though – don't overdo it or you'll look like a Christmas tree! Alternatively, add a streak of colour to your hair, wear coloured mascara and paint your lips in bright or dark red or pink. Bold colours suit your style and your attitude.

You may be a mixture. I am both dramatic and a natural dresser. I love my jeans but I like the quirkiness of a fantastic belt or bag to wear with them. You only have to look at my hair and eye-wear to know that I'm no shrinking violet and that my appearance is pretty *dramatic*. I also love heels and wouldn't be seen dead in trainers unless I'm going to the gym. I could never be an overall *natural* as I can't go out without makeup and my hair done (in fact I can't even sit in the house without both being done), so a definite no-no. Although I can also wear tailored pieces, and look pretty good in a pencil skirt, I opt for trousers because I move very quickly and a tight skirt prevents me from doing so. This *classic* category tends to come into play when dress needs to be appropriate for the occasion, corporate seminars for instance, rather than being my everyday choice. Even then, I'd probably go with Vivienne Westwood as my designer of choice because there is an element of drama in her creations. What I definitely am not is *romantic* or *creative* and every time I've tried to wear something along those lines, I've looked ridiculous. See how it works?

What I would stress is that as you get older, and if you are also an extreme style personality, you may need to tone it down a little. Otherwise you could look eccentric or really frumpy. A good rule of thumb is 80% timeless and 20% trend. This will keep you looking youthful and fashionable without being a fashion victim or a dowdy frump.

My way of doing this is by teaming a great jacket and shirt (both timeless) with skinny jeans or a waistcoat (both trendy). Alternatively, a simple knit dress (timeless) with coloured shoes and tights (trendy).

Using the information gleaned so far, together with your three key descriptors, please answer the following:

STEP 4

What can you do to dress in a more authentic manner? Could you introduce something new to update your look? Which garments can you dispose of because they are alien to your nature?

....

....

....

....

HOME IS WHERE THE HEART IS

If you're still unclear about what your style consists of, take a look at your home. A person's interior décor can often represent the real them.

My home tends to be quite colourful but minimalist. There is no wallpaper, just painted walls. No chintz or frills or flounces. Every room has one eye-catching feature - an unusual painting or an elegant chair. I tend to spend money on the basics, such as a leather suite, and they will be in neutral tones. The accessories will provide any colour. This has the added advantage of making it easy to change the look of the room without spending too much money.

The essence of my home reflects the essential style elements of my dress sense, which is dramatic but easy to live with (sporty). I never wear much jewellery, just a statement piece that will be very different. My clothes are colourful but never frilly or flouncy. My look is quite understated but bold, just like my house.

One of my clients has a beautiful, modern and airy home. All surfaces and walls are white. The only colour comes from some fabulous artwork that she has painted herself. She had contacted me because she had lost sight of her identity and had no concept of what would suit her, now she was older. Her clothes – black, black and more black were often shapeless with no charm or charisma. Once she had realised that her own style preferences existed, albeit within her home, she could transfer the guidelines into her wardrobe. She now dresses in light neutrals, using bright jewellery and lipstick as her colour accents. She sparkles and looks radiant.

So have a fresh look at your own home. What does it say about you? If you are not living in a home that suits your personal taste at this present time, imagine one that would and carry out the exercise using this as your template.

GETTING THE BALANCE RIGHT

How many times do you look in the wardrobe and you just don't have anything to wear? Most of us wear a mere 20% of our wardrobe 80% of the time, which is pretty shocking really. Have you also discovered that when your budget is non existent you find clothes that are a 'must have' but a special occasion outfit is never forthcoming when you're actively looking?

As human beings, we are multi dimensional and so is our day-to-day existence. The various roles we play of mother, breadwinner, aunt, grandma, friend, partner and so on require different types of clothes. Many occasions also call for completely different attire. A balanced wardrobe requires clothes that can serve us for all aspects of our life.

To find out if your wardrobe is working for you, do the following exercise.

Take a piece of paper and draw two circles.

Using the circle as a pie chart, divide it into sections proportionate to the different areas of your life (excluding sleeping time). For instance, 40% may be work, 25% gym, 15% socialising, 10% gardening, 10% slobbing around the house and so on.

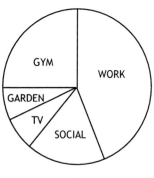

In the second circle, do the same thing with the clothes you own. For example, 20% of your clothes are suits, 10% are jeans, 30% sweaters and so on.

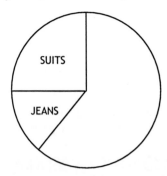

Now compare the results. Do they marry up or has one area totally dominated your wardrobe? Ask yourself why that might be. What are you hanging onto? What are you trying to avoid? If it does tally, well done, you've got it just right.

Using all the information you learned about yourself, complete the next step.

STEP 5

Are your clothes appropriate for your personality, your style preferences and your lifestyle? Do your clothes reflect the image that you want to project – at work and in your social life? Have you got the balance right between work and play? What changes do you need to make?

....

....

....

Some of us crave a different outfit every day, and there is nothing I can say to help you pare down to essentials if you are an accumulator by nature. But if you want clothes that really work, choose colours that co-ordinate so they can be mixed and matched to create a number of outfits to suit all occasions. Use belts, jewellery, hats, hosiery and sunglasses so you can create a myriad of looks.

As the Greek Philosopher, Epicetus once said, "Know first who you are and then adorn yourself accordingly."

WORDS OF WISDOM

✓ Always have your adjectives in mind when you dress.

✓ Your style preference is crucial when successfully buying clothes.

✓ Walk around in any new purchase before you buy and make sure it really loves your body, lifestyle and the effect you want to have.

✓ Make sure you are fashionable or at least current in your choices. You are 50 not 80. When you go through your wardrobe, check out the garments you don't wear and see if you can allocate someone else's style preference to them rather than yours. Bet you can.

Knock 'em Dead (Making an Impact!)

"By itself reality per se isn't worth a damn. It's perception that promotes reality to meaning."

JOSEPH BRODSKY

Each one of you has an image whether you actively cultivate one or whether you don't. The way you present yourself to the rest of the world is the way you will be viewed. Whether that view is valid or not is up to you.

All of us make initial judgements about people in seconds – their background, how much they earn, how educated they are and so on. Humans are programmed to believe first what we see rather than what we hear, so our reference in this process centres round the visual. What we actually say only accounts for very little (7%) of what people think about us. Non-verbal signals, body language, eye contact, confidence, height, weight, colouring, clothing, hairstyles and accessories account for a massive 93%, of which 55% concentrates on our visual appearance alone.

Your image therefore is crucial in terms of your career, an interview, a first date or any event that's important to you.

In the corporate world, this is known as The Spiral of Success. When you look good, you feel good and your self-esteem increases. In turn, this will enable you to project yourself with more conviction and confidence. Others are drawn to you, so you are likely to gain more positive responses from work associates, family, friends and even strangers. From a business stance you are more likely to gain trust and respect. The result – a positive impact on your relationships and, ultimately, your bottom line.

As 90% of our bodies are covered by clothes, it would seem logical to dress in the best way possible. This book should be helping you to do just that. It will give you the chance to look at the basics in an unthreatening way. It will tell you things your best friend might not. It will help you to understand what really suits you, what to wear and when to wear it. If you know you look good, it is one less thing to worry about, so you can focus on the things that really matter to you, whether that be a new career or a new date or looking tremendous at an important function.

Remember, just because something suited you years ago, does not mean your outfit is still appropriate today. A dated look can be interpreted as 'behind the times' in the workplace (and in the dating arena), so if you're not nearing the proverbial glass ceiling and still want to get there, perhaps you should look at your clothing with a critical eye. The same applies to those of you running your own businesses.

Remaining authentic and true to yourself is fundamental to your success. Your 'self' is what you are all about. Understanding how to acquire an image that conveys your true essence to the people around you is the critical factor.

However, there are other factors to take into consideration when dressing in a business environment:

APPROPRIATENESS

Your attire must be appropriate for the occasion – that's a given. You must also take into account your audience and their expectations, your objectives, your industry's culture and the situation itself. Sounds complicated but it's not. Let me give you an example. You would not expect to find a tattooed waitress, with multiple piercings and shoddy clothing serving you in a very upmarket restaurant. If you did, how would you feel about your experience, the establishment and its treatment of its customers? Let down? Not living up to its reputation? You bet.

One of my clients is a Personal Life Coach. She had only just started in her new profession, after leaving the banking world. She couldn't understand why she her client list was dwindling. Checking out her attire, it became obvious. She was wearing the same outfit she would have worn previously to the bank. The pin-striped look was not appropriate for her new clientele, who needed a much softer image for them to feel comfortable.

Admittedly, there are some professions where you must stick to the rules. In the legal profession, for instance, a court appearance will mean a black suit and white shirt. Whether or not it suits your personal colouring is irrelevant. The industry and its culture take priority.

YOUR 'PERSONAL BRAND'

In the chapter 'Who Are You?', there is an exercise to discover your values and how you utilise them to best effect in your dress. Why is it important? Well, if there are two people applying for the same job or contract, their 'brand' is what will tell them apart. For instance, imagine two women applying for the same role within a company and their CVs are practically identical. If one wears well applied makeup and the other doesn't, it's highly likely that the make up wearer will get the job. Why? Because rightly or wrongly it is perceived that she has made the extra effort. In fact, on the subject of makeup, a woman wearing makeup can expect to earn up to 23% more than her bare-faced sisters.

If you are vying to climb the career ladder or secure a new contract, you are more likely to succeed if your attire is correct. Research by Robert Half suggests that in promotional terms, image counts towards a massive 30% of whether the candidate will get the higher grade role. Only 10% is geared around the ability to do the job and 60% is centred on networking and promoting yourself. The latter cannot be done effectively without a good personal image to begin with.

PERSONAL ATTIRE

Your outfit should suit your physical and mental attributes and your budget, though it is said that you should 'dress for the job you want not the one you're already in'. For more information on these topics, please look at the relevant chapters.

DO YOUR RESEARCH

If you are looking for funding, applying for a new job, presenting to a group and so on, it's essential you do your research beforehand. The banking profession is synonymous with pin-striped suiting, the advertising industry is not. Check what you are expected to wear beforehand.

A client told me of her husband's recent misfortune at being turned down for a loan. He works in advertising and had gone to the bank in his normal 'uniform' of black shirt and black jeans. While perfectly reasonable to wear this type of outfit in the advertising world, the bank didn't quite see it in the same light. Her husband had not given enough thought to who he was meeting, the environment in which they worked and the occasion. He was going to them for money and he needed to dress according to their expectations not his own.

FRAGRANCE

I'm not talking about personal hygiene because I'm assuming none of you have a problem with that. I'm talking about perfume. I've actually stopped wearing it for meetings now. Smell can be associated with memories and the emotions they evoke. Even if your scent isn't overpowering, you don't want to remind someone of somebody they didn't get on with or an ex-lover. Best leave it off if you haven't met with the person before. This could well be a good rule to follow if you're meeting a new date for the first time too.

GROOMING

It goes without saying that you should always be well groomed for an important event. This does not mean wearing nail varnish at all times but it does mean having well kept nails. Hair should be clean and tidy and in a style that suits both you and the situation. A soft look will not work well if you want to come across as smart and decisive. The chapter 'It's Not All Black and White' will help you to choose powerful colour combinations if required.

Make sure your clothes fit properly. A gaping white shirt will not be seen as professional, just slutty. Your shoes and your bag are criteria the business world may use to categorise you. Make sure they are clean, polished and preferably the best quality you can afford. This also applies to your outfit. When we are younger, we can carry off cheaper suiting but as we age, it's more noticeable if a fabric is of a lesser quality or badly tailored.

Also a reminder of something many of us forget – clean your spectacles. There is nothing more distracting than smear marks all over someone's lenses. You end up thinking about cleaning them rather than paying attention to what the wearer is saying.

ETIQUETTE

Learn how to shake hands well if you haven't already. A perfect handshake should meet web-to-web and be firm. Try it out on your friends to check that you are not limp-wristed or crushing bones.

Women are often good at small talk but we're not always good at listening. They say we have two ears and one mouth for a reason, so try to practise using them in this ratio if you have a tendency to butt in or talk when the other person hasn't finished what they were going to say.

BAD HABITS

If you make a bad first impression, it can take 21 further interactions before you change someone's perception of you. Most of us are not lucky enough to get the chance to meet with a key stakeholder that many times so we need to get it right first time.

A person, meeting you for the first time, may not remember what you have said but will remember any bad habits you have up to three months later. This can mean anything from leaving your mobile switched on, constantly flicking your hair, smoking, swearing, drumming your fingers, wearing jangling jewellery, having dirty finger nails and so on. To be really sure, check with your friends. Make sure you don't do something they daren't mention to you.

COMFORT

Last but not least, make sure your attire is comfortable. There is nothing worse than watching someone constantly pulling at the hem of their skirt, or adjusting their belt.

Always try on your outfit at least once before wearing it. Make sure the fit is correct and you feel great in it. Check for pulling across the back of the shoulders, wrinkling when you are seated, or any gaping fastenings. If you haven't worn it for a while, make sure it still fits and that it's in good repair with no loose buttons or unstitched hemlines. If you feel great and know you look the part, it will be one less thing to worry about on the day, which enables you to proceed with the job at hand.

WORDS OF WISDOM

✓ Only buy clothes that suit everything about you.

✓ When trying on something that you're unsure about, ask yourself the following – "does it fit my body, is it comfortable, is it appropriate for the occasion and does it reflect what I want the world to know about me?"

Excuses, Excuses

"Looking good and dressing well is a necessity."

OSCAR WILDE

It's so easy when you get older to make excuses about the way you look. At the end of the day, it is just a cop out.

My mother-in-law, Audrey, is in her 80s. In the summertime she walks to the local lido and swims every day. Her garden is her passion. Not only does it look magnificent but it has the added advantage of keeping her physically in shape. She is not afraid to take holidays on her own and will never be short of someone to talk to. She has always had a sense of style, and reaching her ninth decade has done nothing to alter that view. A long-time wearer of skirts and dresses, she took the plunge a couple of years ago and decided to try out trousers for the first time. A new addition to her wardrobe has now made itself known. She even purchased a pair of jeans – so who says you can be too old to wear them? In her wisdom, she realises the benefits of getting the foundation right. The result - her body looks as shapely today as it did when she was much younger.

If an 80 plus lady has the wherewithal to care about her appearance, then so should you. So no excuses please.

Here is a list of some of the excuses I hear on a regular basis, along with my answers. I hope you find them helpful.

It's not worth dressing up as I have grandchildren/small children and their dirty hands get everywhere.

Wear garments with a pattern. This way the dirt is less likely to show up. If you're still taking the children to school, a coat with a pattern is a great way to look modern without looking mucky and unkempt. Team with dark denim jeans and funky trainers so it becomes practical as well.

My teenage daughter thinks I'm too old to wear modern clothes, so I now live in my tracksuit.

This statement could well say more about your daughter than it does about you. Imagine yourself at her age. How would you feel if your mum was wearing clothes the same as yours? The key is to adapt the trends. If your daughter wears skinny jeans with cropped tops and high heels, wear yours with a boot cut to flatter the legs, and team with a cashmere sweater and a great jacket. You can add a belt or a stunning piece of jewellery. Still modern, but adding your own spin to it makes it suitable for your age.

I don't want to be noticed, so I tend to stick to clothes that cover me up.

Whether you like it or not, you will be noticed. It's better to be noticed for the right reasons than the wrong ones. Understated clothes can still be stylish. Baggy, shapeless clothes that shroud your body cannot. So choose clothes that are not fussy, in fabrics and colours that suit you. Let others notice how lovely you look rather than be seen hiding away in a corner. Check your style personality for clues about how to shop.

I feel really fat so I'll change my
image when I lose the weight.

When you've lost the weight, what are you hoping for? If the answer is to feel confident and look fantastic, why put it off until some future date in time? Select garments that will flatter your body shape and colouring now. Instantly, you'll look and feel so much better. The compliments will flow and others may think you've lost weight already. Getting the foundation garments right is another step you can take. A well-fitted bra can knock off up to a stone. Wearing pattern in the correct scale can also disguise any lumps and bumps.

I never have any money to spend on myself.
All my money goes on my family.

When I hear this, the emergency procedures on an aircraft come to mind. In the case of a potential crash, adults are advised to put on their life jackets and take the oxygen masks before they attend to their children. The premise being that if the adult dies, the children cannot take care of themselves so they too will die. I feel the same way about taking care of your appearance. Do you want your child's role model to be a mum who sacrifices everything, consequently looking dowdy and frumpy? Would you want them to do that for their children? Or would you prefer them to have a healthy belief that mum takes care of herself, looks terrific and of whom they're really proud?

Life is too short to worry about the way I look.
People should take me as I am.

Life is short, there is no doubt about that, but the way you look can affect what happens to you in that lifetime. The impact you make and the confidence you have can all make your life easier to enjoy. Dressing to suit your personality and body shape is as easy, once you know how, as dressing in any old clothes. The difference in results? Enormous.

I don't like my legs, so I live in trousers
and never really feel feminine.

Actually, I'm not a big fan of mine either, though my husband thinks they are my best feature. I too tend to like my trousers but if you team them with a sexy top, you can still look stunning. I do wear skirts and dresses but with patterned or coloured tights and boots. Still looks youthful and I do actually feel very womanly. Make sure the hemline sits on a flattering part of your leg. If you have it bisecting your calf, for instance, the effect will be ruined.

Shoes, of course, can make all the difference. Try walking around in a killer pair of shoes, preferably with a low front and high heel or wedge. Your legs will look amazing and you may change your mind about the way they look. Scholl Footwear sells gel-filled pouches which cushion the balls of your feet so there is really no excuse unless you have a physical problem. Podiatrists now say that totally flat shoes are not good for you. The optimum size heel for your leg and foot health is ½ an inch.

I don't have money to spare on new clothes.

These days you don't need lots of money to look great. Designer labels are now creeping into High Street stores, so you can buy good quality at a really reasonable price. Supermarkets sell cashmere sweaters at a third of the cost you would expect to pay. Spend any money you have on getting the basics right. A flattering coat, boots, a pair of trousers (or a skirt) and a great sweater are your essentials. Base these essentials on a neutral colour theme so everything relates. If you choose a pattern, make sure it has some of the neutral in its mix. If you have a large bust, make sure you don't skimp on buying the correct size bra. Tops and accessories can be picked up for very little cost. Choose wisely and you'll always look stunning.

I don't want to look like mutton dressed as lamb.

You won't if you follow the guidelines in this book. Don't make the mistake of wearing something you looked great in 20 years ago – it just won't work. Mini skirts, really low cut tops and 5" stilettos spring to mind. As a rule of thumb, the shorter your hemline the lower your heel should be. Don't try to squeeze yourself into something that is too small. Sizes vary enormously according to manufacturer, even in the same store. Drop any ego and wear garments that flatter your shape rather than worry about what size is on the label. It is eminently possible to look youthful without looking ridiculous. Look at the trends in the shops and adapt accordingly.

I'm too old to change.

You're never too old to do anything. These days you read about 70-year-old women running marathons, giving birth, writing novels and other such marvellous achievements. In fact many 45-55 year olds are changing everything about their lives. Age is a state of mind. You really are as old as you feel. A change of outfit may well enable you to put the zing back into your life. Move out of your comfort zone by taking small steps – a change of colour, a new piece of jewellery, a pair of great-fitting trousers, a new hairstyle. Once you look into the mirror and see your fabulous reflection, you too may want to change more than just your image. Be curious. There's no failure attached.

I don't have a man around, so why bother?

This is the 21st Century! You don't have to have a man around to want to feel special about yourself. Wise up and smarten up. This kind of attitude, along with its partner, neediness, will certainly ensure no man comes looking for you. Make the most of what you've got and you'll be turning them away.

I want to wear jeans but I'm too old for them to look good.

Not true. There are some styles of jeans that I would definitely steer clear of: those with distressed patterns or sequins on the thigh or bum, dirty and stone washed denim, skinny jeans (unless you are very slim with straight hips and legs) and those with crinkled lines around the crotch. A dark denim pair with a boot cut or a wider straight leg can be really smart as well as flattering and comfortable. If you are curvy, opt for some Lycra in the fabric. Check the back view. Some pocket details are sewn so low that it causes the bum to appear lower than it really is. Your best bet is to choose a pair with as little adornment as possible.

Always sit in jeans before you buy to check there is no gaping at the back of the waist and that they are not too tight across the thighs. Does your tummy spill over the top? If so, opt for a higher rise. The hem should reach your toe crease when you are wearing your choice of footwear. Make sure the opening of your trouser hems can accommodate your footwear. Bulky trainers worn with a narrow leg jean look silly but can look great with a wider boot cut. Never buy jeans that are too large as they often 'give' when you are wearing them. The perfect pair is worth hunting for. Once found, you'll be a convert.

Out With The Old...

"'What shall I wear?' is society's second most frequently asked question. The first is 'Do you really love me?' No matter what one replies to either, it is never accepted as settling the issue."

JUDITH MARTIN

As we get older it's only reasonable to expect that we've collected some baggage along the way. If the baggage has a high emotional content, it can be painful to deal with. It can also affect our future and how we deal with situations that arise and people we meet.

There is widely held ethos that if we de-clutter our lives of the things that are holding us back, we can clear space to allow us to enjoy new and exciting experiences.

A similar idea lies behind a detox plan. The idea is to eliminate, over a short period of time, foods that are toxin related. The resulting benefits are a loss of weight, clearer skin, brighter mind and a more self-confident you. But is this kind of treatment geared only towards what we eat? What if we took the same type of approach to the clothes that hang in our wardrobes? Wouldn't it be fabulous if a fashion detox could give us similar results?

The older we get, the more we tend to get stuck in a fashion rut. Black suits us, baggy feels good on us and those faithful old flatties never let you down. Added to which, ever noticed that however big your wardrobe, the clothes you pick out from it daily only ever seem to shrink.

As we get older, our confidence around what to wear can also shrink. None of us want to look like mutton dressed as lamb, but we don't want to look like our grandmothers either. High Street stores tend to concentrate on 18-year-olds or senior citizens. As we fit into neither camp, it's easy to see why we get confused and end up feeling invisible or ignored.

So if any of this rings true with you, try out the following and get ready for some fantastic compliments. If you can't do this today, make sure you find some time to do it SOON. This is important so please don't procrastinate. Please note, a nice glass of wine seems to help the process.

STEP ONE - SORT OUT YOUR WARDROBE
The following three steps will make sure you only have garments that make you feel wonderful. Just like a detox plan, it's about replacing things that make you look and feel low with those that will energise and brighten your whole being. Don't stop at clothes though, remember your jewellery, shoes and makeup can also benefit from this treatment plan.

If you haven't worn it in two years, then throw it out. There is always a good reason why it's still hanging there and not being worn. If it's an occasion garment such as a ballgown, store it away until you need to wear it again.

Be ruthless. If it's too small don't make the mistake of keeping it until you've lost weight. It will act as a constant reminder that you are now a larger size. Instead, prepare to celebrate any future weight loss by buying something new when you've succeeded.

Get rid of mistakes. If it doesn't make you look (or feel) great, if you're tired of it, if it still has its tags, then return it, sell it, give it to charity or a friend, if it will suit her.

If it has a great deal of sentimentality linked to it but you never wear it, then put it in a box and tuck it under your bed or in the basement. But don't let it take up valuable space in your wardrobe if you don't wear it on a weekly basis. Look at it again in six months and see how you feel about it. If you feel the same, then keep it hidden away. Repeat at regular intervals until you're ready to let it go. Ask yourself why it's so important to keep hold of it. What does it make you think or feel that you don't have now? What's missing from your life?

Make repairs: This can also include dying it if it's the wrong colour, altering the hemline, taking it in at the seams, changing the buttons and so on. If you don't take it to be repaired in one month, then you know you're really not that crazy about it, so throw it out.

The Comfort Factor: Comfy old clothes are OK for slobbing about the house and chilling out. But when it comes to the outside world, comfort does not replace style. Clothes should always make the most of your figure. No reason why you can't combine the two.

There are certain items that must go, whether or not they fit or you think they suit you. For example high-waisted, tapered trousers with pleats; mini skirts; jackets with huge shoulder pads and any garment that would look better on your mother.

On the whole, if you haven't worn something in two years, it needs to go. On the other hand, if you're still madly in love with an older garment, that has worn well, is still stylish and makes you feel special – keep it.

STEP TWO - ORGANISE THE GARMENTS INTO SEPARATE PILES

1. Looks good and fits, or would if it was repaired.
2. Would look great if it fitted.
3. Never looked that great but is almost new.
4. Hasn't been worn for over 2 years.

STEP THREE - KEEP THE FIRST CATEGORY, GET RID OF THE OTHERS

Clothes for the 'no mercy' pile include pleated skirts, kilts, anything flannel especially shirts and certain nightgowns, Logo t-shirts, nylon tracksuits, tapered trousers, gold buttoned double-breasted blazers, big knickers, bulky sweaters if they add on pounds, short shorts, ripped, stone washed or glitzy jeans.

Remember, you can make money by selling 'as new' clothes to a clothing agency. Alternatively, if it has a designer label you could try selling it on eBay.

Already you might find that a great weight has been lifted psychologically. Clearing out clutter is very liberating. To make way for the new you have to clear out the old. It will do you no favours to keep it.

Clothes are all about providing the wearer with confidence. A well-tailored, classic garment, such as a coat, can remain current over a period of more than three years. 'Fashionable' items should be worn for the season only. That's why it's never worth spending too much money on them, but there is no reason why you can't mix with something more upmarket for a 'different' look.

WARDROBE MUST HAVES

✓ **A great pair of jeans.** Whatever your age and weight, jeans are a must. Dress up or down according to the occasion. If you have hips, choose a wider leg (boyfriend style) as they will be more flattering. Petite ladies need to wear them long and a straight leg will suit you the most. Tall and slim? You can wear most styles and you are the only shape that really suits skinny jeans, despite what the TV programmes may say. If you don't believe me, try a pair on see what happens to your hips! Boot cut jeans are now almost a classic as they flatter everyone by balancing out the hip and lengthening the legs. As with all trousers, remember to wear them the correct length. Check the hem - it should reach the crease of the toes of the shoes you are wearing and be aware that you may need different pairs to wear with flatties and high heels. This means checking that the hem opening is wide enough to take the correct footwear. Choose a higher waisted style if you have muffin top (overhanging belly) and look for a high lycra content if you're curvy. Always sit down in them before buying to check the fit at the waist and make sure the pockets flatter your derriere. Dark denim is the best choice as it's more stylish and it slims.

✓ **A white shirt** is a staple that NEVER dates but you must make sure it's perfect for you. Cotton will only look great on women with a small chest and few curves. The fabric is too stiff to accommodate a large bust without pulling and will also hide a small waist unless it's cut really well. Choose fabric with some Lycra woven in if you're curvy and you'll find the stretchiness provides much needed comfort. Team with your jeans, a belt or a great long necklace to jazz up a casual look or with a jacket and trousers to give a more classic feel. Bravissimo sell great tailored shirts to accommodate a larger chest so are worth checking out.

✓ **A fabulous t-shirt.** Choose a good quality fabric that will stand multiple washes. White is great but other colours may suit you more. The shape of the neckline depends on your face shape. The depth of the neckline should be geared to your bustline.

✓ **Little black dress.** Chanel made it famous and it will always stand the test of time. Ring the changes by good use of accessories, shoes and tights or a wrap so it looks different on every occasion. If black isn't your colour, choose an alternative colour that looks chic and stylish rather than a fun and funky hot pink.

✓ **A cashmere sweater.** Every woman's luxurious 'must have'.

✓ **Shoes.** The basics are a plain court with 1-1½" heel and a pair of knee-high boots and/or ankle boots. These will take you anywhere. A wedge sandal for the summer is also a great buy.

✓ **Black trousers** – well cut and flattering. As with your jeans, you can smarten them up or pare them down. There are so many on the market, it's essential to buy only the pair you love or they'll end up at the back of the closet. As with jeans, you will need different pairs to accommodate different heel heights.

✓ **Tuxedo style jacket.** Single breasted, with a medium lapel and a hem that just covers your bottom. This style flatters everyone so how can you not have one in your wardrobe? Change the buttons to revamp.

✓ **An A-line skirt.** As with the jacket, this style suits virtually everyone unless you have a very high hip, in which case you might want a hemline that curves in towards the knees. Choose a pencil skirt if you want a sexier look. The length of your hemline depends on the shape of your legs, how low your bottom is (mine is VERY low), how quickly you move (I've ripped so many seams because I race everywhere, that I've given up wearing them now), who you are meeting and the occasion to which you're wearing it.

✓ **A Tote bag.** A large bag doubles up as a laptop case, an organiser and a fashion accessory. The added bonus is it will also slim you down by making you look smaller. A bold design or metallic leather will add some zing to your outfits.

✓ **Well-fitting underwear.** What's the point in carefully selecting your clothes if they look like a sack of spuds once you're in them? If you haven't been fitted recently, make an appointment soon.

WARDROBE MUST-NOTS

These are items that will add ten years to your age and need to go!

✗ **Short, cropped tops.** Please!

✗ **High-waisted, tapered trousers** with pleats around the waistband - burn them, they will make you look short legged, big-bummed and bulky round the tummy.

✗ **Shoulder pads** in anything, unless very discreet or well tailored.

✗ **Big, baggy t-shirts** with short sleeves ending at bust level. These are for men!

✗ **Shapeless cotton shift dresses** with round neckline and no sleeves – especially if patterned. In fact, anything shapeless needs to go unless you are twig-like. Be ruthless, even though these are making a comeback as I'm writing, which also goes to show fashion is fickle and short lived.

✗ **Ankle length pop socks** which show when you sit down. Please!

✗ **Tapered jeans**, especially in stone wash denim, that stop at the ankle.

✗ **Mini skirts**, especially when worn with short, cropped tops showing cleavage and belly.

✗ **Leather trousers** – unforgiving.

✗ **Double breasted blazers** with gold buttons – will make even the thinnest person look two stone heavier.

Once you've de-cluttered, bear the following in mind.

AIR YOUR CLOTHING

Install a hook on the outside of the door. Use it to air out the clothing you wore before returning it to the wardrobe. Doing this will save you money on dry cleaning. Excessive dry cleaning can ruin a garment, so only use if the item is soiled.

USE A FULL LENGTH MIRROR

Everyone should have a full length mirror. Let me repeat – everyone should have a full length mirror. You'd be surprised how many of my clients don't own one. This is absolutely fundamental, otherwise how can you tell what you look like? Install one on the inside of the wardrobe door, or use a freestanding mirror. You need to see your clothing in its entirety to see if an item is really working for you.

LET THERE BE LIGHT

It is absolutely necessary to have a bright light installed in your wardrobe. You need to see what you have in order to wear it.

STAY ORGANISED

To manage your new collection and to make it easier to combine your existing garments, hang clothes by type. Put your jackets together, your trousers, tops and so on. You'll be amazed how many different combinations you can find. If you prefer, you can also differentiate by colour. Do the same for your boots, shoes and sandals. This should save you time when dressing.

STORAGE

Avoid wire coat hangers as they can ruin the shape of your garments. Buy wood (cedar is best) or wider plastic hangers instead.

Knits should be folded rather than hung on hangers, otherwise they may stretch.

Tailored pieces need padded or wood hangers.

Trousers and skirts should be hung from the waist with clip hangers. If trousers are creased, try hanging them upside down from the hems or invest in a trouser press.

If you are short of space, pack away last season's clothes. Garments should be placed in a dark, dry and well-ventilated part of your home. They need to be protected from insects, dirt and odour.

TAKE CARE OF YOUR SHOES

Take your favourite shoes to be re-heeled and resoled. Get rid of outdated shoes. Nothing can date an outfit faster. Toss any shoe that is uncomfortable. Realise that over the years, your shoe size has changed. Your feet have grown bigger or wider, and they're not going to shrink! Invest in shoe-trees or keep shoes in shoeboxes. Stuff shoes with tissue or newspaper to hold their shape. Take a picture of the shoe and staple it on the box so that you won't have to open every box to find your shoes.

BAGS

If you have spent lots of money on a fabulous bag, make sure you keep it in the cloth bag in which it came. Bang out all the dust and rubbish that's collected in the bottom before packing it with tissue paper to keep its shape intact. Use a clear furniture polish on leather handbags to keep them protected from the elements and to extend their life. You should always rotate your bags and never overload them. Not only is this bad for the bag but also for your shoulders and neck muscles.

MAKE A LIST OF ANY 'GAPS'

Last but not least, take a good look at the garments you have chosen to keep. What is missing? Make a list of essential items such as a jacket or skirt. When you next go shopping, take the list with you and ONLY buy what is on the list – NOTHING MORE!

Take a leaf out of the chic Parisienne's book. They always look stylish because they plan their wardrobe, and their shopping. So instead of buying individual garments on a whim, think about what they will complement in your existing collection. As a rule of thumb, if it doesn't go with three other items, don't buy it.

Dame Helen Mirren goes one step further and only buys something if she can throw something away in its place. Not sure I'm that disciplined but it's a great principle if you can stick to it.

WORDS OF WISDOM

✓ If you're unsure of whether or not to throw something out, store it in a different wardrobe. If you haven't noticed it's gone after six months, you can safely discard.

✓ Why not have a 'swap' party with your friends? It's a great way to exchange clothes that might look better on someone else.

Shop 'til You Drop

"Shopping is better than sex. If you're not satisfied after shopping you can make an exchange for something you really like."

ADRIENNE GUSOFF

Love it or loathe it, shopping for clothes is an essential part of our lives. Unfortunately, mistakes happen and regardless of which camp we fall into we can still end up with a wardrobe of clothes and nothing to wear. Pro-shoppers call it retail therapy. They love it so much that any excuse is a good one to scour the stores. Their credit cards are always at the ready to buy up those 'must-have' items as soon as they hit the shelves. If they lived another 40 years, they wouldn't get round to wearing all the clothes that are scrunched up in the wardrobe fighting for space. The anti-shoppers buy only from necessity. As they hate changing rooms (or can't be bothered to get undressed) it's usually something picked straight from the rail and never actually tried for size. With no idea how to put an outfit together, their wardrobes resemble a jumble sale of hapless, mismatched items.

Frivolous or frugal, to be a great shopper you need to have a plan.

Firstly, make a list of what you actually need. This could be a gap in your wardrobe or something for a special occasion. Write down what you'll be looking for.

Secondly, with these items in mind, think about where you are most likely to find them. Do you need a specialist shop or will the local High Street suffice? Will you require accessories? If so, think about where you can buy them from.

Next – work out how much time you have before you need these clothes? Many of my clients ring me in total panic because they have Ascot, a wedding, or a celebration coming up in the next few days and can't find anything to wear. Events need time to plan.

Book a date in your diary and stick to it.

How much money can you afford to spend? Sticking to your budget is often the hardest task as there are so many other goodies to tempt you.

Take any articles with you that will be worn with the new clothes. High heeled shoes, for instance, if you'll be wearing flatties for the shopping trip. I see so many women buying high-heeled sexy shoes wearing jeans. They can't possibly see how they look on the leg or if they will suit the dress/skirt they're supposed to be worn with. This also applies to specialist lingerie such as a halter-neck or strapless bra.

Last, but not least, be comfortable or you'll never stay the course.

Once you're in the store, armed with the knowledge from the previous chapters, you'll be able to quickly disregard unsuitable choices by looking at the fabric, shape, colour and so on just by scanning the rails. If you're unsure, hold the garment up and check again. If it seems to tick all the boxes, go ahead and try it on for size. Remember, fit is critical but size is not. You need to love it and it needs to love you back by ensuring you look fantastic when you wear it. To check that it's true love, sit down, move your arms above your head and then outstretch them to the front of you, walk around. Check your rear view for any draglines or tightness across the shoulders or bottom. Are the pockets in a flattering position? Is the hem the right length? Does it feel soft and wearable against your skin? Do you feel good even if you don't look at yourself in the mirror? If the clothing passes all these tests you're onto a winner.

A word of caution here. If you have been colour analysed and have been given a book of your most flattering colour swatches, don't hold each one against the fabric to look for an exact match. Fabric textures will change in hue especially if they are patterned, so hold the book away from you. If the exact shade doesn't appear in your booklet, hold the fabric over the entire book and see if it harmonises with the rest of the palette. If it does you can go ahead. Many swatch books are limited to 30 colours but there are millions you can choose from. The idea of the book is to point you in the right direction, to make shopping easier, not a chore. Don't become a slave to it.

It's a well-known fact that changing rooms are harsh places to find yourself in. Garish lights that show up every bulge and give the appearance of cellulite even if you're sure you haven't got it, and the unpleasant saleswoman who sneers when you ask for a larger size or refuses to find it for you, all add up to make it a potentially unpleasant experience. On the other hand, some stores have such flattering mirrors you can't fail to be impressed with how great 'madam' looks. If that's not enough, you feel under obligation to buy since the saleslady has been so helpful.

If this is striking a chord, the solution is to buy online. No pushy saleswomen, no tricky mirrors and you get the chance to try on clothes in a known environment with items you already own. Sure, there is the tedious task of returning them if they don't fit, but it's a small price to pay – isn't it? The alternative is parking, queuing and becoming hot and bothered – not great if you're menopausal OR you could book a session with a personal shopper and have them do all the work.

THE SALES

I've never understood the British mentality for queuing up at some unearthly hour to hunt for a bargain but I know I stand very much alone in this. Unfortunately, this dedication doesn't always pay off. I've lost count of the number of the times I've been back to clients' homes only to find entire wardrobes crammed full of unwearable garments only purchased because they were 'in the sale'. Please don't get sucked in. These days every day is a sale. The reason the clothes are on sale is because no one else bought them and they are now out of date. It's the store's way of getting rid of unwanted stock – that should tell you something straightaway!

If you really must indulge, follow these tips:

- ✓ Don't go to the sales without a shopping list and a budget (that you will stick to of course!)
- ✓ A classic garment that will stand the test of time is a great bargain to find but make sure it's not too old fashioned.

✓ Only buy it if you know for sure it will go with other items in your existing wardrobe.

✓ It must fit properly. However much money you've saved it will not feel great if it doesn't hang properly.

✓ Check sizing labels, as the only bargains I've ever bought were because the garments had been sized incorrectly.

✓ Check any refund policies in the store before you buy.

WORDS OF WISDOM

✓ Don't shop when you're feeling emotional. You'll end up with lots of mistakes.

✓ Learn to think 'outfits' rather than buy individual items.

✓ Always shop with a list of what you want and be strict about the amount of money you're able to spend.

✓ Take any items with you that might form part of the new outfit.

The New Obsession

"It's not what you'd call a figure is it?"

TWIGGY (ON HER FORMER EMACIATED BODY)

TV and magazines seem to be awash with programmes and articles about being super slim. Many use video diaries to follow women and their quest to slim down from a normal size 10/12 to become the new Hollywood must have – size 0 (UK equivalent size 4). Many begin their journeys believing it's only about keeping hunger at bay (the diets often have restricted calorie counts of about 500 per day) but ultimately, the results are far more debilitating. Loss of any form of social life, low blood count, tiredness, depression and guilt are all by-products of this new obsession of ours.

These issues concern me greatly. The average size of a woman in the UK today is a 16. To reduce to a size 4 is just not realistic but there are many who will do whatever it takes, regardless of the risks, to do just that.

As someone who suffered with eating disorders in my formative years, I know just what it's like. I stopped eating because my peers (I was only eleven years of age at the time) were much smaller than I was in both height and weight and I wanted to be like them. My confidence was low at a time when changes in your body are of paramount importance. The more weight I lost, the worse I became. You constantly compare yourself with others, you cannot have a social life that involves any form of eating, you become secretive, you find ways of hiding food at the dinner table, you lie about your weight and wear huge clothes to hide your emaciated body and then there's the guilt. The daily weigh-in balances between euphoria (lost weight) or wracking despair (stayed the same or an increase). It's a prison sentence, eventually leading to solitary confinement as you shut yourself off more and more. Are you happy? No way.

I was lucky. I didn't die and I now have a healthy relationship with both food and exercise and I love my body. However, the eating disorders have left scars. I have muscle wastage due to my body trying desperately to conserve the few calories I allowed it to have. Our wonderful bodies are very clever and realise when the body is in starvation mode. To survive it breaks down large muscle tissue to gain nutrients and much needed fat stores. This was the reason some prisoners of war were found alive when starved in concentration camps. Jane Fonda says in her autobiography that her hip replacement was a direct result of her own eating problems in her youth causing osteoporosis in later life. Some anorexics have large amounts of hair on their bodies. This is another survival mechanism, keeping the body warm when fat stores are depleted.

As we near the menopause, it's vital we keep nutritionally healthy and if this means being a larger size, then so be it. Learn to love this new shape of yours and dress it with respect and adoration. For more information on Eating Disorders, go to *www.b-eat.co.uk*.

Up-to-date, factual information on the menopause can be gained via The British Menopause Society *www.thebms.org.uk*

GREEN IS FOR GO

Earlier in the book I wrote about detoxing your wardrobe to rid yourself of unworthy items that clutter up your space. These days it's in vogue for celebrities to endorse a detox diet to revitalise the body but fasting is an ancient practice and can work wonders if properly supervised.

As I stated earlier, I have done many things in my life which have not served me particularly well but seemed to be OK at the time – excessive sunbathing, heavy smoking, too much alcohol and an unhealthy pattern of eating. I'm amazed that I don't look nearer to 70 than 50, especially when you throw in widowhood at 28 years of age, stress and the fact I was a couch potato into the mix.

Since coming through my eating problems, I've always been interested in good nutrition, but smoking still loomed large in my life. None of my friends and family smoked and I hid it from most of my colleagues, as it certainly didn't fit in with who they thought I was. So when I decided to quit, it was like a massive weight being lifted from my shoulders.

Quitting needed to be easy and it was surprisingly easy, especially for someone who had smoked for over 30 years. My method of choice was acupuncture, which I underwent with a wonderful lady named Ella Keepax. One of the reasons for her success was she looked into the emotional causes behind why I had continued with my habit even though I had moved on in every other area of my life. Once we had discovered what they were, she was able to work with them and I haven't had a craving since. What was strange was that I developed a real hankering for fresh fruit, specifically berries. I'm assuming my body needed lots of vitamin C, as it had been very deprived over the last few decades. The cleansing by acupuncture also affected the rest of my eating patterns and I found myself only wanting fresh food, nothing pre-packaged, microwaved or mass produced in any way.

Being of a curious nature, I decided to look around and investigate what I could do to enhance this fabulous feeling of being healthy. For once in my life I could aspire towards the energetic, slim figure that had always lurked inside and find true pleasure in what I was eating. So out came the books on nutrition, cookery, vegetarianism and so on and I delved into all of them to see what occurred and how I felt.

After some dabbling with macrobiotics (Madonna) PH Balance (Gwyneth Paltrow) and vegetarianism, I came across an article in a Sunday supplement on Raw Food. The chef, Karen Knowler, was local so I decided to give her a ring. As it happened, she was running a weekend course starting the following Saturday so I booked on. I loved the way it made me feel and the energy I had with this type of eating.

So what is Raw Food? Basically, it's based on the premise that heating food causes the molecular structures of a food to change and our bodies do not cope well with it. All food is eaten uncooked, mostly vegan and organic in origin. Green foods play a huge part and that suits me because I love them.

I have always promised myself never to be rigid in my eating again as I have too many painful memories of what it was like to be a social outcast due to my eating problems of the past, so it's unlikely I'll ever be 100% raw.

Leslie Kenton, *www.lesliekenton.com* a wonderful and inspiring woman who has been teaching us about good health for years, advocates 75% raw with grains, lean meat, fish and pulses making up the rest. Delving into these various eating plans, I've come to the conclusion that she is right – at least for me anyway.

I have found a way of eating that really does sustain both my body and the planet and I feel very nourished (there is also very little washing up – a great bonus). I'm also enjoying more water and herb teas, and have reduced my intake of coffee and alcohol, but I haven't cut them out completely as I still enjoy them. Chocolate remains on the menu but more often in the form of cacao nibs, which are my and Gillian McKeith's form of heaven (*www.gillianmckeith.info*).

I'm certainly not advocating that you all become raw foodies but I do urge you to look at your diets and make sure you are eating in a calorie-poor, nutritionally high way. Living on junk food will not help you in the long run and if you are in your 40s and 50s, payback time may come sooner than you realise.

I am not a nutritional expert but if you eat a variety of natural foods in rainbow colours, you are likely to stay healthy. Virtually anything that is green will be of high nutritional value. Orange, red and blue are also good for you and often contain lots of vitamin C. Try to eat these most of the time and certainly on a daily basis. The medical profession advocates five portions of fruit and vegetables per day and if you can stick to that, you're well on your way.

Over-processed, refined foods such as white bread and pasta, those with added salt and sugar or a multitude of chemical names and E numbers should be banned to the dustbin or eaten in moderation. It's common sense that if what you eat remains as close to its natural state as possible, it probably will be better for you, so use whole grains instead.

It makes sense to source organic food, even though it is more expensive, as you know it has not been treated with chemicals and pesticides. The farming of animals brings some horror stories but it's your own choice whether or not you decide to eat meat and fish.

Milk is a strange choice and it's really not meant for human consumption but to nourish calves. I always hated it and my school playtimes were constantly cut short while I struggled with the warm bottles of milk we were forced to imbibe. Luckily, there are alternatives such as soya – good for the menopause – rice and almond milks so I for one am very happy.

If you're unsure of your diet at this time, book a consultation with a nutritionist or read some books. There are plenty out there which give sound advice specifically for our age group and cater for the bodily changes we are (or might be) going through – Leslie Kenton (*www.lesliekenton.com*), Marilyn Glenville (*www.marilynglenville.com*) and Maryon Stewart (*www.askmaryonstewart.com*) are experts on food and its effect on menopause, recommending natural herbs instead of HRT to combat any hormonal imbalances.

Enjoy what you eat and if you remember your grandma's old adage – everything in moderation – you won't go too far wrong.

Ella Keepax BSc Hons Lic Ac MBAcc can be found at 144 Harley Street W1 G7LE Tel: 07787 118931

Karen Knowler can be found at *www.therawfoodcoach.com*

WORDS OF WISDOM

✓ If you're unsure about what to eat, divide your plate into four. Fill one quarter with protein such as lean meat, fish, eggs or pulses, the second quarter with complex carbohydrates such as brown rice or a jacket potato and the other two quarters with lovely fresh vegetables or salad.

✓ If you're unexpectedly tired or bloated, keep a food diary and see if it has a direct link to a food type.

✓ A little bit of what you fancy does you good.

It's All In The Mind
(Exercise For Mind & Body)

"Exercise - you don't have time not to."

ANON

I really was a couch potato at school and the memories of PE still make me shudder. Even now when I walk into a school gymnasium, memories come back to haunt me. So you can take it that I am not one of life's natural exercisers and, in fact, couldn't even touch my toes until about four years ago.

Things have progressed since then and I passed my Fitness Instructor qualification about ten years ago, just to see if I could. It was a 40th Birthday challenge and the hardest thing I've ever done. It did prove though, that you can achieve whatever you put your mind towards – so take note.

I'm not going to write a whole chapter on the pros of exercise and how good it is for us – that's a given. Though you may want to think about the type of exercise you undertake, as it needs to change as we age. Weight bearing exercises are particularly good to prevent the onset of osteoporosis and walking is probably better than running if you have joint problems. Pilates is fantastic if you want to tone up your tummy and have a really strong centre core and better still, you don't need to sweat.

My own exercise of choice is yoga. I like the idea of it being non competitive and how it promotes the union of flexibility and strength. If you've ever participated, you will know that the breath is the most important aspect of a yoga practice. Without it, the class is simply another exercise class not a yoga session. Focussing on the breath not only helps to move valuable oxygen to the blood cells to energise and invigorate but also enables the mind to focus and slow down. For me, this is especially important as it enables my brain to switch off, even if it's only for the duration of the session. The Chinese actually believe that an individual only has a certain number of breaths in their lifetime. If you slow down your breathing, becoming more relaxed, you'll also live longer as you won't use up your quota so quickly.

There are many types of yoga so classes tend not to follow a set format, with the exception of Ashtanga, and you never know what might crop up next. I like this idea of the unexpected (being curious again) as it heightens my enjoyment of the session. With other types of exercise, my physical body has certainly been present in the room but my mind has definitely been outside of it, doing its own thing and reminding me of problems, to-do lists and so on.

One day, while I was struggling in a horrendously challenging yoga pose trying to focus on my breathing but not succeeding very well, my yoga teacher started to talk about the *eight limbs of yoga* which appear in Pantanjali's Yoga-Sutra. Written over 2000 years ago, they act as guidelines to provide a structure to both one's yoga practice and one's daily life. The first limb is called *yamas or* yoga don'ts.

The first of the yamas is *Ahimsa* – do no harm. Generally speaking it means the day-to-day practice of non-violence. So far so good. I don't beat up old people, or harm animals so I felt I could ignore with this one. But could I? Or you?

My yoga teacher was trying to explain that holding an uncomfortable position for too long causes actual harm. The body doesn't like being under stress and the next day there will be a price to pay with sore muscles and the like. As yoga is non-competitive, why would we want to put ourselves through this? Why aren't we happy to allow the body to show us what it can and cannot do? After all, as the yoga teacher pointed out, this is the only body we will have in this lifetime, so why abuse it?

You may not practice yoga but I often see and hear how the majority of women do not practice *ahimsa* when it concerns themselves. Non-violence doesn't just apply to what you do but what you think and what you say, both to others and to yourself.

Check if you do any of the following on a regular basis:

✗ Compare your body negatively to those of other women (or celebrities).

✗ Hate looking in the mirror.

✗ Spend ages focusing on every line and wrinkle.

✗ Dislike part or parts of your body and/or face.

✗ Think about cosmetic surgery as a way to make you feel better about yourself.

✗ Deny yourself food so you can squeeze into a small size or 'comfort eat' on junk food.

✗ Buy loads of clothes but never feel that any of them make you look wonderful.

✗ Think if only I had longer legs, a prettier face, blonder hair etc I could be so much more successful, happier, confident and so on.

✗ Put off doing something worthwhile until you are thinner.

✗ Yearn for a time when you were younger, slimmer, blonder.

✗ Forget you are a unique person in your own right who is blessed with talents, skills and attributes, both physical and psychological, that no-one else shares.

If you are doing any of the above then you are being cruel to someone who is *very* important – *you!*

I can't change your behaviour overnight – it's too ingrained. It doesn't help that we Brits have a habit of self-deprecation. 'It's not cricket' to be too proud of ourselves. No one likes a bighead! I would, however, like you to consider the following:

From now on buy only clothes that you *love*. It could be the colour, the fabric, the style, the fit – hopefully it will be all four. Do not buy anything that you feel lukewarm about. This applies to your underwear, your bag, your scarf – everything. The purchases don't have to be expensive, just gorgeous.

Remember size is just a number. Fit is everything. If the size label bothers you, cut it out. Do NOT go into spasms of guilt because you think you have put on weight. A garment is often cut to fit a particular model (usually a size 10) and then scaled up or down to provide other sizes. That's why some brands favour a curvier woman and some do not. If the model does not share your proportions or your overall shape, the garment won't fit properly. End of story.

The future is uncertain. While I don't want to bring gloomy thoughts into the equation, it's true that you never know what might happen to your body in the future. Celebrate what it can do for you now. Love it, pamper it, nourish it, be kind to it, after all it is part of the whole you. One day what you have right now might seem like a godsend. In yoga, it is said that you can only really live at this present moment in time. Make sure you make the most of yours by enjoying your body, your clothes and your life right now.

Get into the habit of thinking nice, pleasant thoughts. Every time you meet someone, notice what is good about them and, if the situation allows, give them a compliment. It must be heart-felt – we all know when someone isn't being genuine – and observe how gratified they are. You've probably made their day. Once you get into the habit, you'll start to notice how many compliments come your way too. Accept them graciously and say a big 'thank you' in return.

Oh and by the way, yoga will also give you great posture. You can looks pounds slimmer without even trying!

The British Wheel of Yoga will list details of qualified instructors in your area. *www.bwy.org.uk*

WORDS OF WISDOM

✓ Only take part in a particular sport or exercise if you enjoy it. If you don't enjoy the gym, find something else to do instead. Try salsa dancing, gardening, walking the dog or golf. The important thing is to keep active.

✓ Don't fret if you're not very good to start with. As long as you enjoy it, you'll improve. Pat yourself on the back for what you can do now.

✓ Buy appropriate kit that you love to wear. This will motivate you to attend every session.

That Will Do Nicely
(Plastic Is Accepted Here)

"Nature gives you the face you have at twenty; it's up to you to merit the face you have at fifty."

COCO CHANEL

You can often tell the age of someone by the way they walk or the way they hold themselves but more often than not, it is their face that gives them away.

I had always believed that being authentic meant making the most of yourself 'naturally' regardless of how miserable you were feeling inside. This all changed about a year ago when I met up with a friend of mine for lunch. She is the least vain person I know and about ten years younger than me. Over lunch, she confessed that she had made an appointment to have blepharoplasty (eye bag removal). I was really shocked as firstly, I hadn't even noticed that she had any problems with her eyes but secondly because my friend just wasn't the 'type'. I suppose I had categorised women who had surgery as some kind of wannabee celeb/footballer's wife types with huge orbed breasts and wind-tunnel expressions on their faces. I hadn't actually stopped to think that ordinary women might choose to go through with something like this. It made me think, especially as I had had so many problems with my own baggy eyes. She had struck a chord deep within me.

A couple of months later, we went to lunch again. What a transformation. Not in her actual face – to be honest I couldn't really see too much of a difference – but in her whole persona. Here was someone who was completely happy and confident, effervescent in fact. So much so, she virtually kissed her reflection in every shop window we passed. The operation had most certainly changed her life, her outlook, her self-esteem and she was radiant.

I couldn't stop thinking about her and suddenly everywhere I turned I was bumping into others who had gone under the knife with amazing results. Clients opened up to me about breast reductions, a tummy tuck, eye bag removal and a breast uplift – none for total vanity but because they were so miserable and/or in pain. I realised that I had been very 'judgmental' and 'superior' of those who had undergone treatment without being totally aware of their reasons for doing so.

In the end I discussed what I was thinking to my husband. He knew how I felt about my eye bags and most days trod on eggshells not knowing how to respond to, "how do my eyes look today?"

To give you some idea, the left eye had three bags one on top of another and the right had two. On a bad day, these reached my cheekbones. The condition, I later found out, does have a name – festooning. My spectacles, which should have been my style statement, had become my mask. I dreaded taking them off to read or to speak to a client, in fact some days the bags were visible beneath the bottom of my frames. I would cancel yoga or exercise classes (where wear contacts) if my eyes looked too bad (I also have sinus problems which caused even more puffiness) as I couldn't bear to see myself in the mirror. Bear in mind too that I had come through an eating disorder and had completed the exercise in 'Mind Over Matter' very successfully for the rest of my body. Despite years of angst over how I looked, I had come to a place where I was as happy as I could be, except for my eyes which had been my best feature when I was young. Friends and relatives had always remarked on how they could always tell what I was thinking and how I was feeling by my eyes. Yes, your eyes are the windows to your soul but not if you don't want anyone to look into them. Although confident on the surface, my feelings about my facial appearance were at an all time low.

It dawned on me that cosmetic surgery could provide the solution but I felt a mass of emotions: guilt, fear, fraudulence and shame at the very thought of going through with it. If the emotional side wasn't bad enough, on the physical side I scar very badly so was worried that I might end up worse as a result.

In the end, I made an appointment to see a specialist – Mr Ahmad – at my local hospital. I decided that I would just go for a chat as I could always say 'no'. He was the surgeon who had carried out the operation on my friend and had a highly respected reputation in his field. He put my mind at ease and gave me the options, also noting that, "I had a youthful figure and outlook but my eyes were letting me down by ageing me" – how true.

I'll cut the story short but I went to see him more than once for reassurance and even the day before my operation was due, I was on the phone to his secretary in tears, still feeling emotionally wretched about what I was about to do. Amanda made me feel much better by really listening to me and what I was saying. I realised there was nothing else I could do to rid myself of the eye bags and if I truly thought I was worth maintaining, why shouldn't I do it?

That was a year ago now and yes, it has made a huge difference to the way I feel about myself. Has anyone noticed? I don't think so, only in respect of my being happier and more confident. Mr Ahmad did a good job and my eyes look totally natural. I can honestly say that I look less tired now, even when I don't sleep through the night, than I did when I was completely fresh and awake in the past. Was it worth it? Absolutely. Do I want anymore? The answer is 'no'. I now feel balanced in the way I appear to myself and those around me. Before, I was an old face on a younger body and it felt totally wrong. Now my face matches the rest of me.

Here are some guidelines for you if you too want to go down this route:

✓ Make sure you choose a surgeon that appears on the General Medical Council register and check his/her qualifications thoroughly. Mr Ahmad performs his operations in hospitals and I felt safer than if it was in a private clinic. The nurses I saw beforehand all rated him as top class and this did a lot to alleviate my worries.

✓ Ask for photographs of before and after, what could go wrong, possible side effects, how long the procedure will take, recovery time (mine was three weeks in total but for the first week you cannot see anything at all, so you need someone to take care of you) and any possible scarring – this was a real concern for me as I have two keloid scars from other non cosmetic operations.

✓ Find out what you need to do before and after the operation to help you to a fast and safe recovery.

✓ Find out if this is permanent or will you need to have another operation in years to come.

✓ Ask for referrals if possible.

WORDS OF WISDOM

✓ No operation is risk-free so assess whether you can live with the risks.

✓ Don't feel guilty if you decide to go ahead. If this is the only way, you have every right to use it to enhance and unleash your real self.

✓ Go through the exercises in the 'Mind Over Matter' chapter first. Cosmetic Surgery is not a quick fix for any emotional problems you may have.

✓ Tariq Ahmad MA FRCS(Plast) can be contacted via his wonderful secretary, Amanda Oliver, on 01223 864678

The Sassy Woman Within

"The only real elegance is in the mind. If you've got that, the rest really follows from it."

DIANA VREELAND

As we approach our 50s, many of us are reluctant to look more modern for a number of reasons. We are scared to shop in places like Top Shop or H&M as we feel too old. Worse still, we don't want to wear what our daughters are wearing (and vice versa).

Life begins at 40, so they say, but it can be scary knowing that middle age is here right now another 10 years on. Many of us may feel like we've lost our identity. What are we supposed to look like at now we are 50 or fast approaching it?

If the following ring a bell, you're not alone:

- ☐ To be thought of as 'mutton dressed as lamb' is horrifying.
- ☐ We feel we look older so we wear an older person's clothes.
- ☐ We believe that chic, classic tailoring will see us through. Actually, sometimes it will, but on the wrong person it can be very ageing – (think 'power' dressing, shoulder pads and scarves of the 1980s).
- ☐ We don't want to look like our mothers so we stay in a time warp of too tight dresses and mini skirts or clothes that remind us of happier times.

- ☐ We are in a rut and don't know how to get out of it.

- ☐ It's easier not to bother so we don't go out or make any effort at all.

If you fit into any of these categories, then read on. Here are my top tips for the SASSY woman to look modern and stylish right NOW.

FOUNDATION IS KEY

Wearing the correct bra in the right size is critical. Get yourself measured, regularly. A bra's shelf life is four months maximum so don't feel you need to make up reasons to buy a new one. If your tum's your problem area, try control underwear on those occasions where you want to look slim and sexy. Otherwise, buy knickers that support you. There is nothing worse than seeing someone's cellulite through the fabric of their trousers or a very visible panty line.

FLATTER YOUR FIGURE

Understand what fabrics and shapes suit you best. Ignore this basic style principle at your peril. Contoured shapes need fabrics that skim over the curves. Angular shapes need more structure to enhance the straight lines. Cover up your problem areas and concentrate on making the most of your assets – you now know what they are - and show them off to dazzling effect.

HIDE THE FLESH

Less is more. To be alluring, we need to have some mystery. At our age, our skin is not that of a young girl so be discreet.

ADAPT THE TRENDS

Look at what's in fashion in the magazines and High Street stores. Instead of following slavishly, take the main idea and adapt to your own shape. Remember 80% timeless teamed with 20% trendy is a good combination to follow. A pair of jeans teamed with a cashmere sweater and a fantastic jacket will always look modern and stylish. Stick to boot cut for a more flattering effect.

ACCESSORISE

Too many accessories can give you the 'Christmas Tree' effect. When you get older, less is often more, especially if you are petite. Choose wisely and pick just one great accessory to add some dramatic impact. A large, unusual piece of jewellery, a fabulous handbag, or a great belt can all look terrific. If you wear glasses, make sure they have your name on them. Don't wear unsuitable frames as it's the first thing someone will notice.

BE TRUE TO YOUR PERSONALITY

Be authentic in your dress. There is nothing more draining than trying to be someone else. Use your style preferences, your essence and your intentions to help you choose what to wear and how to wear it.

WEAR THE CORRECT SIZE

There is no actual standardisation of sizing of women's clothing in the UK, so all of us will have at least three different sizes in our wardrobe, and that's not counting garments for fat/thin days. If you wear clothes that are too small, you will look bigger. If you wear clothes that are too big, you'll be swamped.

WEAR FLATTERING COLOURS

Especially near to your face. Warm skins need warm tones like olives, golds and browns to enhance your glow. Cool skins need cool tones like blue and pink to flatter the skin. You can sometimes go a little warmer if you are 'medium' colouring or on the borderline of warm/cool as it will help you look younger but experiment and gauge reactions before changing everything. The wrong colour can drain and add years. The same goes for hair, so choose your stylist with care.

STAND UP STRAIGHT

Poor posture can ruin any outfit. If you've made all this effort, make sure you can carry it off to your best advantage by standing tall. In yoga, they refer to the 'bandhas' and in Pilates, the 'core' or 'powerhouse'. This is the place in your body where you need to concentrate your effort. Place two fingers widthways below your navel and pull it in. Make sure you can also breathe. If done regularly, it will strengthen your abdominals and make you appear leaner. Imagine a string being pulled from the top of your head. Move into this position and pull your shoulders down and back. You should be able to feel the difference straightaway – perfect posture and a younger, thinner you.

EXPERIMENT

Don't be afraid to experiment (think of my word curious again). If you've had the same look for years, make the transition easier by adding small changes until you become comfortable and confident with the new look you. Swap trousers for the occasional skirt, try a belt around your waist or your hips and see what happens. Make use of mail order catalogues and try clothes on at home, where the mirrors don't lie. This also gives you the opportunity to combine new purchases with your existing wardrobe.

SHOP WISELY

You now know which items to spend money on and which can be bought cheaply. You are also aware of the staples that make up your wardrobe so you can add to your basics rather than buying a garment that doesn't go with anything else. Always take a shopping list and don't detract from it. Think in terms of outfits not garments. Only go to sales if you know for sure there is something worth buying. Otherwise give them a miss. After all, it is only stock that the shop no longer wants and there's always a reason for that.

LOVE YOUR CLOTHES

When you are trying on clothes in a shop, walk around in the changing rooms, sit down and see what happens. Has the garment creased? Does it restrict you in any way? Is it comfortable as well as flattering? Do you LOVE it? Only buy clothes that you love if they love you back (sounds like good advice for most relationships).

DE-CLUTTER REGULARLY

There's nothing more liberating than throwing out the old. Make way for new clothes and new ideas. Clearing space in your home is said to provide more clear space in your head.

USE THE ART OF DISGUISE

If you're feeling under the weather, use the tricks of the trade. Use large spectacles or sunglasses to hide dark circles or puffiness around the eyes, wear a flattering colour around your face, divert attention by clever use of jewellery, apply your favourite lipstick and cheer yourself up with a spray of a fabulous fragrance.

If all else fails, wear brightly coloured shoes. I can't count the number of times I've been rescued by my lovely red shoes when I've had a bad face day. How does it work? You have been taught that the eye sees a bright colour first. Where you wear it on your body makes no difference. By putting on my trusty (and sexy) red shoes, all eyes go to the floor rather than my puffy face. I've even had admiring glances and comments on a crowded Victoria Line platform at the height of rush hour. It works – really it does.

FIND A GREAT TAILOR

In the USA, women think nothing of having their clothes altered. We are more reluctant here. Don't be. Great tailoring can make transform an outfit.

BE GRATEFUL

Thank your body for doing its job. It's the only one you have so treat it with respect and care.

LOVE YOUR LOOK AND LIVE YOUR LIFE

Be proud of what you have achieved. Live your life with passion and zest for all things, not just your clothes. Dressing well is just the first step on the road to confidence and success. Enjoy each day and make the most of every opportunity that comes your way. Celebrate your age, pamper yourself, eat wonderful food, keep active and learn to accept the inevitable compliments – as you'll be receiving lots of them from now on – be radiant in your magnificence and stay curious about everything that comes your way. You can't help but remain youthful and attractive to everyone you meet. As Christian Dior once said, *"Zest is the secret of all beauty. There is no beauty that is attractive without zest."*

What Next?

"I have a dream."

MARTIN LUTHER KING

Now that you are well dressed, confident, healthy and SASSY, where do you go to next? You have the power to do whatever you want and that can be quite daunting. If you have a dream this might be the best time of your life to follow its path. If you don't do it now you may never have the chance again.

When I worked in the corporate field, which I did for many, many years, I was issued every year with objectives and targets that I needed to achieve. Although I invariably succeeded, at times it was hard to take ownership as they had been set by someone else. Even now, the words *objectives, targets* and *goals* leave me cold.

A much better and more fun way of planning your life is now available and I have used it many times with my clients. It's easy to do and fills you with such incredible joy that you'll probably never use the old system again.

You can do it two different ways but if you do both, you have every chance of succeeding, however far out it seems to be at this present time.

YOUR PERFECT LIFE

Firstly, take some time to sit and ponder about what your perfect life might look like. It's important to think BIG and don't worry about how you're going to get there. You may want to split it into sections, such as family, career, finances, health, romance or whatever is important to you. Or you may just want to focus on one thing such as finding a new career, a new partner or a life abroad.

Take your journal and write down what your perfect life looks like. It's critical that you write as though you are living it now, so it must be in the present tense e.g. "I am married to the most wonderful man," rather than, "I will meet a fabulous man and we will get married."

As you are writing, feel every sentence in your blood. It should excite you. If it doesn't, go back to it and analyse what's wrong. Perhaps you're not thinking big enough or perhaps it would impact on something or someone else that's important to you. Change it as necessary. Keep writing until you've exhausted yourself. This is your Vision Story.

At the moment, exciting as it is, it's just words. To make it even more powerful you need to add some visuals. From this day on, every time you see a picture in a magazine or book that reflects your Vision Story, cut it out and paste it into a book. Keep it near to you and try and look at it every day. This will keep the vision alive. I know it sounds mad but it really does work. I'm not the only one to have found my perfect house, my dream career and a fabulous husband by creating my annual vision.

If writing isn't your thing, you can create a Vision Board. Cut out pictures that reflect your chosen life and stick them onto a large piece of paper. If you can, paste your highest aspirations at the top of the paper and your foundations at the bottom. It's not essential but it helps. Put this somewhere in easy view so you can look at it daily.

The only thing that is important is that you truly feel alive when you read your story and look at your pictures. This is your perfect life so don't skimp on it.

When you Feel *Fab* at 50, the world truly is your oyster.

"Our deepest fear is not that we are inadequate. Our deepest fear is that we are powerful beyond measure. It is our light, not our darkness that most frightens us. We ask ourselves 'Who am I to be brilliant, gorgeous, talented, fabulous?' Actually, who are you not to be?"

MARIANNE WILLIAMSON

10 Things You May Not Know About Sue Donnelly

1. My heroine as a child was Lady Penelope from Thunderbirds. I have FAB 1 sitting in my office as a reminder of how I would like my own personal Parker. In the meantime, I'm training my husband for the role!
2. I love green foods and a meal without them is sadly lacking.
3. I sing tenor in a choral society – with the men – and I used to play the trombone.
4. I was widowed at 28 and I married again at 45. I have 2 step children and 3 nieces.
5. When I was a child I used to spend my time dressing Sindy and Barbie and writing stories. Funny how life turns out!
6. I read Theology at university but left to work for Thomas Cook, where I spent the next 21 years.
7. Jazz is my favourite music, especially the great female vocalists such as Ella Fitzgerald, Billie Holliday and Cleo Laine. I have also seen Barbra Streisand perform live twice.
8. I am the only Fashion Feng Shui® practitioner in the UK and one of a handful of image professionals qualified both sides of the Atlantic. I'm also the President of The Federation of Image Consultants, a qualified life coach and trainer.
9. Apart from shopping, my favourite pastime is reading and I would work in a library if they allowed you to talk. I also love Test Match Cricket - especially if England win!
10. At 50 I am happier than I've ever been as I'm doing exactly what I want to do.

About Sue Donnelly

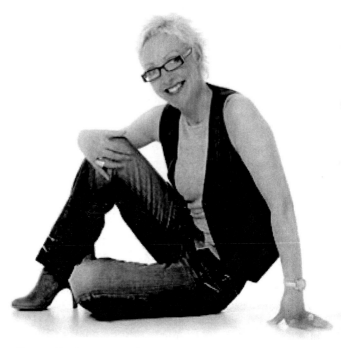

Sue Donnelly is an Image Coach who epitomises the new breed of 50 year old. She loves her work, her life and her body but understands that reaching 'middle age' can be very scary for a lot of women. Sue's passion and friendly nature enables her to assist her clients to find their own uniqueness and a style of dress that reflects their inner values and personality. Not only does this elevate self-esteem and confidence but helps them to get what they want out of life, whether that's a new man, a change of career or a rejuvenated thirst for living. She has been featured in numerous national magazines and newspapers and has been invited to appear on prime time television. She is President of The Federation of Image Consultants, an Image Consultant trainer for Aston+Hayes and the only certified Fashion Feng Shui® practitioner in the UK. She is also one of a handful of people qualified in image on both sides of the Atlantic. Giving to the community is important and Sue works as a volunteer for the breast cancer charity, Look Good Feel Better. As a qualified life coach, trainer and workshop facilitator, Sue has the skills and the rapport to help women look and feel good about themselves in an authentic way. Her other books, 'The 30/20 Makeover', 'Does My Belly Look Big In This?' and 'Heading South?' are available from *www.amazon.co.uk*

For more information on her workshops or to book a private session, please contact Sue by:

Email: sue@feelfabat50.com
Website: www.feelfabat50.com

FEELING FAB AT 50?

If not, you might want to consider spending some valuable time with Sue in person.

If you...

- Feel like you have lost your identity
- Have no clue what 'middle age' dressing looks like
- Don't know how to make the most of what you've got
- Own shed loads of clothes but have nothing to wear
- Think it's all too much trouble

...then help is at hand.

There's no 360 degree mirrors, no baring your flesh and no horrid comments. You'll have a totally transformational experience with someone who really cares – about you. And, she knows her stuff!

Don't wait too long as Sue is in demand.

Speak to her and find out how she can help you on **0845 123 5107** or email her on *sue@feelfabat50.com*

For events, workshops or to read her blog visit *www.feelfabat50.com*

Printed in the United States
124639LV00001B/15/P

9 781905 430345